ROSEN METHOD

ROSEN METHOD

*An Approach to Wholeness
and Well-Being
Through the Body*

ELAINE L. MAYLAND, Ph.D.

Foreword by Marion Rosen, P.T.

52
STONE
PRESS
Santa Cruz, California
&
Santa Fe, New Mexico

Rosen Method

52 Stone Press
433 Rider Ridge Road
Santa Cruz, CA 95065
Phone: 831-425-3509
E-mail: cwabit1@yahoo.com

Edited by Jeanie C. Williams
Cover Design by Richard Harris
Book Design by BlueGlassHeart Productions
Photograph of Elaine L. Mayland by Theresa Garcia

Cover painting by Elaine L. Mayland,
Untitled, oil on canvas, 24 x 36, 1972.

Printed in the United States of America

Library of Congress Cataloging-in-Publication Data
Mayland, Elaine Loomis
Rosen Method: An Approach to Wholeness & Well-Being Through the Body
p.   cm.
ISBN 0-9773796-0-4
I. Title
2005

To the Ruby Slippers

ACKNOWLEDGEMENTS

Documenting Marion Rosen's work initially took me over five years. This edition is the result of another twenty years' work and development of Rosen Method. I would like to thank Marion for her generosity in giving of herself toward this end. I would also like to thank my colleagues, clients and students who have shared in this journey with me.

The section on physiological perspectives was co-authored by Jill S. Kuykendall, Physical Therapist and Certified Rosen Method practitioner. Jill taught classes in anatomy and physiology to students of Rosen Method and to others before moving away.

Paul Flavell, Edmund White and my sister, Louise England, provided invaluable editorial assistance and personal support on the first edition. Theresa Garcia and Zach Howe assisted with proofreading on this edition. Jeanie Williams has worked closely with me in editing the 20th anniversary edition. We have changed the language in several places so that it better serves this work and our readers, and have stayed as close as possible to the original intent of the first edition.

TABLE OF CONTENTS

PREFACE

Marion Rosen's central concern is that we continually seek ways to bring ourselves closer and closer to truth. Truth is, for Marion, a personal quality. The truth she values is the personal expression of individual essence.

Her life's work is a nearly perfect mirror of that belief. Each of her convictions stems from a natural willingness to consider myriad possibilities. These possibilities have been the creatively drawn questions she posed for herself and then struggled to answer. She modestly refuses to credit herself with any special abilities. But in fact she is remarkably quick at recognizing and nurturing creativity wherever she finds it. A major part of the work at the Rosen Institute is the development of a methodology to increase openness and creativity.

When students attend the workshops or classes of the various training centers, they are required both to give and receive sessions. This practice imprints the concept of bodywork as a two-way process between practitioner and client, not a one-way intervention. Marion herself has pursued her own growth throughout her entire professional life. Only by embracing and participating in their own growth through practice can students expect to understand her perspective.

Students will recognize certain basic assumptions and operating premises that Rosen Method shares with other forms of bodywork. This work seeks neither to ignore such similarities nor to underscore them. Marion Rosen came to her principles through her own process and experience and her method of developing one idea upon another is very much a part of what she wants her students to receive from the training.

On Apprenticeship

The training and certification program is completed through an apprenticeship. One cannot become a certified practitioner of Rosen Method any other way. This book was written to help the beginning student by providing a context for understanding the practical work in which he/she will be engaged.

Students should know at the outset that they have embarked on a course of study as likely to raise questions as to answer them. Rosen Method is an approach to opening a broad-based, experientially determined, alternative perspective on the human condition—nothing more and nothing less. It is dynamic, constantly evolving and open-ended.

An apprenticeship is not an easy mode of training for students accustomed to didactic study of facts and techniques. The content of the material determines the method. Students' sensitivities and skills are sharpened only through commitment to self-knowledge and exploration. Periodic evaluations are made by both student and instructors, but in the larger sense every day is an examination—a test of self and others.

The work of Rosen Method practitioners demands intimacy and self-disclosure. To be able to lead others to the trust called for, one must have first-hand experience of the process. Trust, intimacy and self-disclosure are constantly reciprocated and the training center strives to provide a supportive atmosphere.

The apprenticeship creates the opportunity to learn by transmission.

The teacher transmits by her own example to her students both the content and the essence of the teaching. This process goes beyond providing information. It is like the measles: you catch them by being around someone who has them.

When practitioner and client connect on a meaningful level in a session, the journey toward wellness or wholeness can begin. The student must show progress toward an increased sense of self before beginning to assist another on the same journey. Accordingly, the first phase of training is focused on the student's ability to gain personal insight and openness. During the second phase and internship, students come to realize that training has no end, that the work of being true to oneself is a lifelong process and unique to each individual.

This book is only an introduction to the work. Actual understanding of the work lies in the experience of it, which cannot be adequately described. A description can merely suggest the possibilities.

I was inspired to write this book as a teaching aid when the usefulness of a written source of information for students became clear. This book represents my effort to verbalize the non-verbal substance of this deep and subtle work. Since Rosen work is not a "fix-it" method, this book is not a "how to" guide. It is a reference for students of Rosen Method who wish to have the verbal content of the classroom teaching reiterated. I hope it will also be useful and interesting to readers who are not involved in the training.

On Confidentiality

Confidentiality is essential to any intimate work done professionally. Rosen Method is certainly no exception. Central to the work is the idea that we have all learned to restrict and repress ourselves, both emotionally and muscularly. Through Rosen Method, areas of holding are contacted and whatever has been held has the possibility to surface. The Rosen practitioner must create and maintain a space where material that has been held down, or in or against, can surface and be re-experienced or remembered in an atmosphere of safety, trust and acceptance.

A Note on Terminology and Case Material

For the sake of clarity, brevity and readability, the practitioner is called "she" and the client "he" throughout the text, excepting some case material. This terminology does not mean that only women are practitioners and men are clients, of course.

Case material is used anecdotally in much the same way that quotations from Marion Rosen are used. All indented quotations in the text are Marion Rosen's words.

Case descriptions have been altered to preserve clients' anonymity without distorting the essence of what took place. There may, however, be some distortion by abbreviation of the case presentations. While the process is sometimes as dramatic as suggested by the brief presentations, most clients come for many sessions over a long time, even when change is slow, even almost imperceptible. Accounts of those periods have been omitted from the case descriptions.

This book is the result of my experience with Rosen Method and as an intimate friend of Marion Rosen since 1979. This book is the expression of my desire to describe Marion Rosen's work so that others can share in the deep personal meaning it has for me. As her work grew over the years out of her individual treatment of clients, she paid little attention to the systematic recording of what she was doing. As far as she knew, it had no important connection with anyone else's work.

I have cooperated closely with her on the development of this book. Her innocence about her accomplishment within the field of body/mind work and the fact that it was part of a larger scheme continues to amaze me. Her response is simply that truth is truth, in any appearance. She remains excited to find that others have come to conclusions similar to hers.

This book presents Marion's teaching as it is, leaving my observations, opinions and points of view out of it as much as possible, with the exception of the final chapter and the recently added Afterword.

FOREWORD

On the 20th anniversary release of this book by my friend, colleague and senior Rosen Method teacher, I can say with strong conviction that the way the work is presented here is as true to the nature of the work as when it was first written in 1985. I still believe that the heart of the work is in the experience of it—which cannot be fully described because it is an individual process. Some aspects of the work can be talked about, however, and that is the purpose of this book.

I have come to understand that the body is a repository for all of the person's experiences, conscious and unconscious. I wish everyone in the world could experience Rosen Method because it has such a profound impact on people. I always say when someone comes to a lecture, they have already committed to being part of a circle that goes on because you cannot go back to unconsciousness once you've become conscious. Once you have an experience, it is yours. You cannot undo knowing. I often hear from people who have worked with my students and my student's students. There are many people who have been touched by this work all over the world now.

I can recall talking with a very sophisticated audience about this work nearly 15 years ago. I could see a glow in their faces; to me it looked like their eyes were precious stones starting to glow; and the glow was slowly spreading over their whole body. As I spoke further about this work, I noticed that the people in the audience were becoming more and more beautiful. Lines in their faces began to disappear, backs and shoulders were straightening and from their sharing I sensed that they had gotten what it was that I was trying to talk with them about. What was it that came out of me that they could see and understand? I noticed that something touched those sophisticated individuals in my audience in a way that transformed the way they were. They showed themselves to me—and to each other. This book is an attempt to recreate that experience of exchange and learning.

Very often when I work on people, they remind me of flowers that have not yet bloomed. A flower bush looks very different before the first buds appear. And so it is with the body that is closed and does not reveal anything of its life and beauty. The tension in the body presents a picture of lifelessness and as we put our hands on those lifeless parts, the body slowly starts to open like the bud that opens into a blossom full of color and beauty. The human being is capable of emerging from the nondescript mass before us into full color and aliveness. This is the place of possibility from the person we think we are to the person we truly are. From here, there is a choice. As the breath starts moving through the body, its outline changes into something alive; its opening has the same effect as the flowering bud. The person becomes the beautiful being that was hidden away under a stern outside. This process never fails to touch me in my deepest being and so I open up towards the being under my hands. The contact thus created is one of deepest connection and trust and seems to open channels of love on both sides.

You cannot hurry a flowering bud to open to its full bloom. It opens when it is ready to open. It is the same with our work: we may suspect there is a beautiful being under our hands, but all we can do is patiently wait while we put our hands on the held muscles. Our joy is to witness this process, slowly bringing it into the awareness of the person we are working with.

FOREWORD

After so many years, what I find most rewarding about this work is the incredible possibility that people have and that we are allowed to witness. The goal of this work is to bring you to a place where there is no barrier between your internal experience and your external expression of yourself. You do not oppose the universe, but become part of the universe. Letting this happen is the attitude of surrender and trust. This book shows us the way to that place of possibility and choice that is within all of us.

—Marion Rosen, P.T.

1

BIOGRAPHY OF MARION ROSEN

It takes a long time to grow young. —Pablo Picasso

There was a very awful day in Germany, the 9th of November, 1938, when the Nazis went around to Jews' houses and would smash the houses and some of the men were taken to concentration camps. That was a very, very frightening evening. The night before this happened, I had a dream and there was a big, big sky and there was a woman's face; a very lovely woman filled the whole sky and she said, "Don't worry, I'll look after you." And that was all, that was the end of the dream. I just let myself be directed wherever it went, wherever the way opened up.
—Marion Rosen

Marion's European Beginnings

Marion Rosen was born in Nuremberg, Germany in 1914. Her father's import-export business prospered in the years immediately following World War I and the family lived in moderate affluence. Marion was the third of four children; she had an older brother and sister and a younger sister.

In Marion's memories, her mother was a great collector of people. She had a fondness for music and musicians, art and artists, ideas and philosophers, learning and professors, commerce and shopkeepers and people "from the street." She became friends with those who could expand her interests; she often entertained them at home.

Marion, as a small child, was sickly, suffering from recurrent sore throats and bouts of asthma. As she grew older, her health improved. By age fourteen she was already five feet nine inches tall and enjoyed swimming, horseback riding, hiking, bicycling, skiing and above all, dancing. She had a burning desire to become a professional dancer but was told that she could not because she was too tall. She remembers her childhood fondly as carefree and fun-filled, with the single exception of her embarrassment about her height.

The political climate in Germany changed drastically during Marion's teen-age years. Despite her mother's atypical lifestyle, she was rearing Marion and her sisters "to marry rich men and have children." Marion's father once said he had enough money so that none of his children would have to work. Matters in Germany worsened after Hitler's election and it became obvious that Marion and her sisters would have to support themselves after all. By the end of her teen-age years, Marion had tried her hand at typing, shorthand, cooking, embroidery and housework but wasn't good at any of them. She had a talent for languages and had thought she might become an interpreter, but she was not admitted to university because she was Jewish. This barrier was confusing to her because, although Jewish by birth, she had been brought up Lutheran.

In Marion's words:

> I tried different things to do because it was obvious that I had to leave Germany and I would have to earn a living. I couldn't think for the life of me how. I was brought up not to wash my own stockings or if my bicycle needed air in the tires, I would have a man do it for me. I was really not a very practical person.
>
> I was on a hike in the mountains with some friends and we stayed there overnight. When I came home in the morning, my mother was laying down because she had broken her ankle. She greeted me and said, "I have found a person who will train you."
>
> She had in mind the woman she met when she broke her ankle and who had helped her until the doctor came. Usually I wouldn't have listened to her, thinking it was just another one of her fanciful ideas, but I said, "Who?"
>
> She said, "Well, there are two people here and one is a Mrs. Lederer who lives in New York. She does breathing and relaxation work with Karen Horney and she could employ you if you wanted to go over there. Her friend is here with her, a Mrs. Heyer, who lives in Munich who said she would like to meet you and if the two of you click, she might like to train you!"
>
> A few minutes later I met both women and took an immediate liking to them. Mrs. Heyer asked me if I would like to train with her. I said yes and that was all.

Lucy Heyer was a masseuse, a dancer, the wife of Dr. Gustav Heyer (a colleague and former student of Dr. Carl Jung) and a student of Elsa Gindler. Elsa Gindler was the principal investigator then working on the integration of physical and personal development. She is generally considered the forerunner or "grandmother" of today's breathing and relaxation techniques.

The Heyers were part of a group of people in Munich using massage, breathwork and relaxation in conjunction with psychoanalysis as practiced by Jung and others. The group discovered that by synthesizing their several disciplines, the treatment time for psychoanalysis could often be dramatically reduced. Patients came to Dr. Heyer from all over Germany when it became known he was achieving results in far less time than other psychiatrists. It was this fertile, experimental clinical setting that Marion entered to begin her two-year apprenticeship with Lucy Heyer.

Although the Heyers were by then divorced, they still worked together. Psychoanalysis was left to Dr. Heyer and his colleagues; Mrs. Heyer and Marion conducted the breathing and massage sessions in near silence.

Marion remembers, "Sometimes the patients would cry and sometimes they would have pain or lose their pain, but always it was the analyst who did the talking."

Marion once interrupted her two-year study with Lucy Heyer to go for six months to the Tavistock Clinic in London, where her brother was completing his psychiatric residency. She obtained work at the clinic and began to put into practice the techniques she had studied in Germany and again, the patients she treated lost their symptoms. However, the London doctors, who were finding their patients improving much more quickly than they expected, had no approach for dealing with the asymptomatic patient within the psychoanalytic framework. Further, since Marion was naïve about promoting her work at the clinic, she felt herself a failure and returned to Germany to complete her training with Mrs. Heyer, who considered Marion her most gifted pupil.

By the time she finished her training with Mrs. Heyer, Marion's parents had fled Germany for England. Her older sister had married and gone to Switzerland. Marion and her younger sister went to Sweden to wait for American visas.

This waiting period was a difficult time, as Marion had only a letter of introduction from Lucy Heyer, no legal status and was living with her sister in the home of a friend of their father. Marion's sister obtained a work permit and the two of them lived on the sister's small earnings. Marion needed to occupy her time while waiting for her visa. Her visa took two years in coming. Marion remembers:

> First I went to somebody who was teaching dance and asked if I could watch. I said I could massage and maybe do some exchange. As luck would have it, the dance teacher had an incredibly sore ankle. I gave her three treatments and it improved greatly. She was interested in me after that. Then I gave her a treatment for lumbago on the afternoon before she had an evening performance. From then on I was allowed to come and go as I pleased at the dancing school. I spent a lot of time there watching the dancers.

Dance was not the only pursuit that enhanced her understanding of the human body during the months she was in Sweden. She took a formal course in physical therapy. Lucy Heyer's teachings were supported and validated for Marion by the progressive nature of Swedish physical culture work.

> I heard about physical therapy training and went to see the man in charge. He was very sympathetic to my plight and interested in my work with Mrs. Heyer. He said I was welcome to join the class. I spoke very little Swedish so took my notes in German. About a quarter of the way through the course, my notes became Swedish! He let me graduate with the class and wrote a letter saying I had done so. I knew there were some things he appreciated from my earlier work with Mrs. Heyer. The class was very interesting to me and that was my first formal physical therapy training.

As part of the program, Marion observed various operations, watching hip replacements, bunionectomies and vertebral disc and brain surgeries. Thus, in two years' time, under difficult circumstances, Marion had gained exposure to some of the most progressive and important work going on in the field.

Marion received her visa at last and she decided to take the road not previously taken: to go to New York and work with the woman she had met in her mother's parlor in Nuremberg, Gertrude Lederer and Lederer's colleague, Karen Horney. By that time the Germans had invaded Norway and the only route to America was through Eastern Europe, Russia and Japan. Her sister's visa did not come through, so Marion sailed alone for the United States from Japan at age twenty-four, landing in San Francisco instead of New York. Marion's sister remained in Sweden, married and reared a family there.

Settling in the United States

After seeing San Francisco and Berkeley, Marion decided to make her home there. She lived with a German family in Berkeley and did occasional work as a physical therapist. She found the early 1940's atmosphere in Berkeley particularly stimulating and, much like her mother, she began to seek out interesting people who were accomplished in their fields.

A young woman physician who was familiar with Marion's work, along with the woman's husband who was a physicist, felt Marion had the potential to become a physician. They encouraged her to begin a pre-med course at the University of California, Berkeley. One can only imagine what contemporary students must have thought of the tall young woman with little money and a German accent in the man's world of pre-med studies on the Berkeley campus of 1944. She managed to maintain a B-minus average, not high enough for admission to medical school.

Besides attending school, Marion was working the "swing shift" as a physical therapist at Kaiser Hospital in Richmond, treating injured workers from the Kaiser shipyards. After the war, there was a tremendous need for physical therapists for the wounded. Marion learned of a tuition-free program at the Mayo Clinic in Minnesota that trained people for the relatively new (in the U.S.) field of physical therapy. She enrolled and because she was an advanced student, was accelerated through the course to graduate in six months.

She returned to Berkeley and resumed work at the Kaiser Hospital in Richmond, California but found she had little zest for the hospital environment. The staff was overworked and had insufficient time to give to individual patients. She often treated 40 patients a day.

Soon, she and her former supervisor at Kaiser formed a partnership and went into private practice in physical therapy, an innovative step for that time. She changed her name from Marion *Rosenfeld* to Marion *Rosen* at this point as there was another physical therapist practicing nearby under a very similar name. She and her partner opened an office in the basement of a physicians' office building in Oakland. There, Marion continued to treat patients for over thirty years.

Marion was married for a short time and in 1949 she gave birth to a daughter. Marion's original business partner retired soon after. Marion then joined forces with another woman for a short time and then with Gritta Green. Marion's reputation grew slowly but steadily. Her office was near the offices of several orthopedists whose patients often required long-term physical therapy. Physicians making referrals to Marion soon learned the value of her opinion and treatment. Many patients were sent with the simple orders, "Do what you think is best."

In her daughter, Marion found herself with a living laboratory for observation of the development of the human body and psyche. Marion's strong opinions about the effects of child rearing practices upon the free and natural movement of the body stem from her own experiences as a parent.

Through patients who came to her with problems of physical origins, Marion learned of the potential for the body to heal itself. They taught her a great deal about the nature of the will to be well as a factor in maintaining body movement and health. She noticed that patients who talked with her about the events of their lives at the time of their accident or injury were the ones who recovered most quickly. She became convinced of the connection between mind and body and became increasingly successful in treating patients with psychosomatic illnesses—those with origins in emotional stress and withholding.

Marion continued developing her techniques and theories in this setting for thirty-five years. Despite her expertise and with an ever-widening reputation and roster of successes, she herself lacked the conviction that she had developed any special process. She knew only that she was a caring physical therapist and also a very busy single mother at a time when there was far less support for that role than there is today.

Some of Marion's friends came to her occasionally for treatment of tight muscles or tension-related aches and pains. One of them asked Marion for something to do to prevent the aches and pains. From this simple request Marion began her movement classes in 1956. She used the range of motion tests used in physical therapy as exercises, set them to music and had the women do them once a week to keep their joints lubricated and the muscles moving freely and fully.

She held her first class in the living room of one of her students. The original five students were soon joined by others, making it necessary to move to a larger space. As attendance and interest increased, a second class was started. These two classes, taught by Marion, remained in continuous operation for several decades, with many of the original students in attendance.

As her daughter matured, Marion found more time to consider the achievement of her life's work. A patient brought her the key to an important life change. A woman whom Marion had been treating with little result appeared upon her therapy table in a suddenly much improved condition. Marion asked what had brought about the change. The woman told her that she had just taken a weekend course with Werner Erhard called "Mind Dynamics." Marion had never heard of the training but sought it out, so impressed was she with the change in her patient.

Marion credits the Erhard seminar with giving her the confidence and perspective to seek new opportunities in her life and to take credit for work well done. In her words:

> I had become aware of knowing really much more than I had ever let out. So I began to say things to my patients and it seemed to make a great difference. This is how I reawakened

an interest in the verbal part of my work and really when it began in earnest.

As Marion began to open up to the possibilities of discussing her patients' conditions with them, she began to realize that she did indeed have something to teach and so began her training of students by apprenticeship.

At present, Marion is actively involved in guiding her students in Berkeley and abroad. She has come to accept the role of leader, a difficult one for her. She remains a student as well. Marion continually seeks to understand more fully the mystery of the mind-body relationship and to support and foster the value of self-knowledge and self-acceptance.

2

THEORETICAL BASIS

If you bring forth what is within you
what you bring forth will save you.
If you do not bring forth what is within you
what you do not bring forth will destroy you.
— Jesus, Book of Thomas, *Gnostic Gospels*

If you do not let yourself be the way you are,
your body cannot function. The same is true for the
emotions. The only way you can be who you are is
through surrender and self-acceptance.

— Marion Rosen

Rosen Method flows directly from the practice of physical therapy. It evolved through years of clinical practice of physical therapy apart from other intellectual, academic and philosophical influences. Until the establishment of the Rosen Institute, little effort was made to describe systematically the operating principles and ideas underlying the method. It was fiercely pragmatic and relied solely on the evidence of clinical experience.

Only after Marion Rosen accepted the challenge of teaching did she have to transform her accumulated knowledge from its tacit, intuitive state to a more literal and transmissible one.

Part of the difficulty of discussing the philosophy of Rosen Method is its very simplicity. When asked to explain the philosophical basis of her work, Marion replied:

> Naturally, as we come into this world we are not beings that hold back; we are beings that are open. When we are born, when we start getting up and we start moving, we move according to very elementary mechanical and physiological rules. The body works when you move and behaves according to these rules. No effort to it. But we put something in the body that makes it more difficult to move and then we freeze in this position. Why does this happen? There is always something that seems to necessitate a certain way of non-movement, non-living in a certain way. And every time something stimulates it again, we hold it again. We hold a little bit more. And we have forgotten that this is what we do. These elements are partly in the physical body and partly in our emotional being. And in the end, probably in our spiritual attainment.

The underlying concerns of the approach are transpersonal and transcending, based on our common experience as embodied beings. The method is based on the premise that a natural and optimal state of human physical and psychic strength exists. Rosen Method aims at obtaining or regaining this optimal state where the full range of possibilities for expression and authentic, spontaneous behavior exist. As such, Rosen Method is a pathway to self-awareness and self-acceptance.

Rosen Method treats mind and body as an interactive unit. The body does not have meaning as an object. Body is imbued with mind and mind is embodied. The Rosen practitioner acknowledges the potential power of all psychic elements of which some knowledge exists—the unconscious, the parapsychological and so on—but places particular emphasis on the role of the emotions, because it is the emotions that have emerged, again and again, in her work. All of her technique is similarly rooted in her clients' experiences. Her methods are those that have proven to have practical application for her clients.

Because mind and body are inextricably linked, Rosen practitioners connect with one through the other. Their particular talent is affecting the mind and body by contact with the body. The point of entry to the system is through the body.

In bodywork, it is easy to assume that some manipulation is being done to the client; however, the Rosen Method practitioner is a facilitator of awareness and change, not the creator of it. The practitioner observes the places in the client's body where chronic tension is held and where free movement of the breath does not occur. Through contact with the tight muscles, often experienced as barriers, the practitioner meets the holding at its own level, as though reminding the muscle that it is holding and that it has the inherent possibility of relaxing. The practitioner's hands follow the client's process; thereby inviting awareness, and relaxation can then become an option.

As the process unfolds, practitioner and client may talk about what is happening in the body and in the client's experience. Chronic muscular tension is the bodily expression of repressed earlier feelings associated with experiences that were too difficult to manage at the time they occurred.

When the practitioner contacts a client's tight muscles, and his awareness makes it possible for the tension to relax, the experience of the earlier event is sometimes felt. From this insight, the tension pattern that the client developed to survive the experience often relaxes and the client has the possibility of experiencing his authentic or true self. This information is never new to the client. What one learns as true in life is that which one has already experienced but has not accepted, has not acknowledged, or has forgotten. There is no new knowledge, simply a new knowing.

The Rosen Method practitioner pays close attention to the breath and breathing. A change in the body/mind relationship will occur or can be detected via the breath. In Rosen Method, the breath is an indicator of change in the body/mind and is the intersection between conscious and unconscious processes.

The diaphragm, the major muscle involved in breathing, is innervated by both the voluntary and autonomic nervous systems. Because of this dual innervation, attention can be and is paid to the "unconscious" or "natural" breath. When a client relaxes and stops performing or "doing" his breathing, the practitioner watches his breath for changes. She looks for changes in the natural or unperformed breath that indicate that the client has made a connection with repressed emotion linked to tension in the muscle being touched. When the practitioner observes this change from her external perspective, she can verbalize her observation and give the client an opportunity to connect this change with his inner experience.

The breath is the intersection between mind and body. The breath is the most readily available channel for tuning into the body/mind dialogue. The breath is doubly interesting and valuable because it is both a voluntary and involuntary action. Voluntary breathing is linked to conscious activity, involuntary breathing to unconscious activity.

Marion Rosen's apprenticeship with Lucy Heyer initiated her concern and interest in the breath. Heyer had studied with Elsa Gindler and both were in agreement that breathing, although not completely understood, was an important area of investigation for bodywork theory and practice. This interest and conviction has become central to Rosen Method.

When the diaphragm is tight, the body does not function at its best. As the major muscle for breathing, the diaphragm is essential to a state of well-being. Its free, full movement can only be allowed; it cannot be performed. Holding in the diaphragm represents a state of "doingness" in the body, a state with an emotional counterpart.

The client's unconscious processes shape the body. In the socialization process most people adopt roles, play games, wear masks, put up façades and put barriers in the form of muscular tension between themselves and others. They feel or believe that their genuine or authentic self is at risk somehow. The roles, games, masks, barriers and façades develop subtly in response to spoken and unspoken demands and pressures, become structured in the body and require muscular tension to maintain.

Our bodies and our characters are shaped by the familial and social forces at work as we mature. The attitudes taken on as a result are carried and expressed in the body, forming habit patterns that are embodied as rigidity and restricted movement.

For example, a baby has no trouble at all expressing feelings spontaneously, usually by crying. As the baby grows, he or she gets the message that crying is not permitted or valued as a means of expression. When the tears come, the child stops crying by tightening the muscles of the neck and chest. When the urge to cry comes again, the child tightens the neck and chest and refrains from crying. Later on, the tightening of the neck and chest muscles becomes habitual and the child no longer feels the feelings that would make him or her cry. Repression is complete and the child grows into an adult with a chronic stiff neck and non-movable chest and shoulders.

One may have a chronically tense body without becoming severely disabled. The most damaging long-term effect of unregarded bodily tensions is the capping of the individual's potential for self-actualization. Self-actualization can result from allowing chronic tensions or habitual holdings to soften, with a resulting shift towards the authentic expression of emotions as they occur. Rosen Method practitioners can feel, see and trace the movement of the client's breath into formerly held areas.

No value or importance is placed by the Rosen practitioner on the trauma in one's life that made it necessary at the time to create a barrier or chronic muscle tension. A barrier is a barrier. It doesn't matter if it was formed because the child didn't get a jelly sandwich when wanted or because of a major loss. The practitioner contacts the barrier, not the experience itself. But the client may become aware of the emotion attached to the barrier and thereby gain access to a new way of being in the world.

The reason for the holding is unimportant to the practice of Rosen Method. What is important is to acknowledge the need to repress in the first place, the chronic muscular tension required to maintain the holding pattern, and the examination of whether that need still exists.

When the client experiences the original need for the barrier, he may be surprised by what he finds. Sometimes, however, the relaxation happens without the content or story coming into consciousness. Even if the content does not surface, the client still experiences relaxation and the possibility for choice. If, however, a story is available along with the relaxation of the muscles, the client is given the opportunity to say what it is. The event becomes real if it can be shared and the original need to repress loses its impact. As the habit of repression is thereby challenged, future repression is less likely.

The underlying basis of Rosen Method is well expressed by the following quotation:

> *If you bring forth what is within you*
> *what you bring forth will save you.*
> *If you do not bring forth what is within you*
> *what you do not bring forth will destroy you.*
> —Jesus, Book of Thomas, *Gnostic Gospels*

3

PHYSIOLOGICAL PERSPECTIVE

Co-authored with Jill S. Kuykendall, R.P.T.

The dictionary definition of "health" is, roughly speaking, "free from sickness." However, we could look at it as something more than that. According to Shambhala tradition, people are basically and intrinsically good; or in Buddhist terms, people inherently possess Buddha-nature. That is, from these points of view, health is intrinsic. Health is. This attitude is one of being fundamentally wholesome, with body and mind synchronized in a state of being which is indestructible and good. This attitude is not recommended exclusively for the patients, or for the helpers or doctors. It can be adopted mutually because intrinsic goodness is always present in any interaction of one human being with another.

—Chogyam Trungpa

Our work applies itself to the person. The system can be corrected through the person. We contribute to the healing powers of the person so that the body can reverse the aberration that brought about the illness. We listen and support the person in their change. The body is an outside manifestation of an internal state of being.

—Marion Rosen

The Body in Space

The Rosen practitioner works with a simple yet powerful model of the body's occupation of space. As a three-dimensional entity, the body has height, width and depth. The degree to which the body's dimensions occupy its potential space determines how much room is available for the body to move and to breathe. Thus, the ability to participate in the environment is optimal when we are as tall and as wide and as deep as we can be.

The body is the base of sensation. Along with touch, pain, temperature and positional sense, feelings and thoughts have physical correlates that register in the body. A person's consciousness of these physical sensations and of the feelings and thoughts associated with them is also determined by his/her occupancy of the proper height, depth and width.

A primary aim of Rosen work is to allow the body to assume the shape and size that it has within it to become. Usually what prevents the body from actualizing this shape and size is its pattern of chronic muscle tension. The muscle tension and the breathing pattern, which have been programmed by automatic, habitual responses, are the practitioner's source of information about the client.

The Rosen practitioner's point of entry into the body/mind system is the musculature and breathing of the physical body. She uses musculature and breath as guides to the emotions and essence of the client. Rosen Method begins here, on the physical level and advances into work with emotions and language.

Action of the Muscles

Muscle is capable of contraction and relaxation. At the cellular level, its structures overlap, to permit contraction of the muscle while it performs a function. Once the function or the activity is complete, the muscle relaxes and regains its original, optimal length. The optimal length of a muscle is the length that allows the muscle to be maximally relaxed while retaining its ability to maximally contract.

If part or all of the muscle is constantly contracted, with no relaxation and lengthening phase, its potential has been partially or completely spent. The muscle has become less dynamically functional. It will hold the body part static and its ability to facilitate an action or a function is reduced, thereby diminishing the dynamic nature of the body: its ability to move.

A typical muscle is attached to two bones in such a way that when it contracts the bones move around a joint and closer together. If the muscle is chronically contracted, the bones may be statically positioned and the joint is, to varying degrees, immobilized and compressed by the constant contraction. The immobilizing of the joint is the opposite result of the dynamic concept of muscle contraction. Instead of functioning and moving as intended, that part of the body becomes less spacious, less mobile and less functional.

Such chronic muscle tension contributes to rigid posture and limited movement patterns that can precipitate or cause discomfort. The body may not indicate anything is wrong until immobilization and pressure of the joint surfaces against each other, over time, results in pain. Attempting to move an immobilized joint creates the sensation of resistance and possibly pain.

The body should be receptive, mobile and responsive. Areas that are unreceptive, immobile, or unresponsive are usually bound by chronic muscle tension. Voluntary attempts to relax accomplish some change. After voluntary attempts to relax, the residual tension is the result of involuntary or unconscious realms of neurological stimulation.

The person whose body is bound by muscle tension experiences the world with restricted options to move and to register sensation. Sometimes desired activities are affected. For example, the neck is capable of several natural motions—forward, back, side to side and in circles. But if neck musculature is tight, movement is limited. Activities that otherwise would be facilitated by a mobile neck are stressful.

The body is capable of a multitude of movements, but generally only a small percentage is used in daily activities. For example, an individual gets into a habit of waving in a certain way, or nodding in a certain way, or gesturing in limited ways. One does not use all the movements that a body is capable of. Thus, one's experience of and exchange with the environment is limited. There are hundreds of thousands of words in the English language, but some individuals limit their vocabulary to as few as 200 of them, making full self-expression difficult. This limitation is analogous to the limitation of body movements as a result of chronically held muscles.

The body is a vehicle for many possible experiences. The purpose of Rosen work is to increase awareness in the body, acknowledge the present actuality of tensions and limitations and to introduce the possibility of more space and movement. These changes mean changing the habit patterns of the body. Apart from our thinking habit patterns, we have somatic habit patterns. When a habit pattern is changed, different neurological information is transmitted from the periphery of the body to the central nervous system.

When more options are created by allowing the body to be used in a new way, less habitual pathways are used. This exchange of new for old pathways is the disintegrating/reintegrating effect of Rosen work on the body. Change comes about not as a result of the Rosen worker doing something to the client in an intrusive way but by providing a supporting and caring environment for something new to happen through verbal and physical contact with the holding.

Rosen work may bring about various kinds of changes in the body. A muscle may quiver before softening. Circulation may be enhanced, bringing warmth and color to the area. The rhythm and depth of the breath may change. These results indicate a change from established habits. The shift may be simple, yet it may bring a profound response, both physically and emotionally. The shift also has an impact on the immune system.

The immune system and all other body systems are influenced by relaxation, as relaxation brings the body close to agreement with its natural function, just as chronic tension took it away from its natural function. Relaxation supports normal functioning, which was there before disease occurred. Disease is a process often triggered by *dis-ease* in the body.

Physical function depends on one's state of being. Subtle signs of *dis-ease* are given by the body prior to a shift into disease. The practitioner calls attention to the areas of *dis-ease*, inviting clients' awareness, which can result in a change of habits or lifestyle that will enable a shift back toward wellness. Becoming well again is facilitated by relaxation, for then the body's self-healing mechanisms may function without muscular impairment.

The Diaphragm and Breathing

The functioning of the diaphragm is a key element in reading the body. It acts as a "barometer" for how an individual is in the world. The diaphragm differs from other muscles. Most muscles have two ends with the tendon at either end attaching to the bone, but the diaphragm is a round, dome-like muscle that attaches in a circular fashion to the bottom of the thorax. It attaches to the tip of the sternum and around the edge of the lower six pairs of ribs. It attaches in the back to the twelfth thoracic vertebra and to the first three lumbar vertebrae by two long tendons. These are called the crurae and they help to anchor the diaphragm posteriorly.

The diaphragm appears during the fourth week of gestation. It initially develops at the level of other neck structures, thereby sharing innervation with neck and upper shoulder structures. As the embryo develops, the diaphragm descends to its point of attachment and brings its neurological supply from higher up in the spinal column in the form of the phrenic nerve. The center of the diaphragm is called the central tendon; it is acted upon when the diaphragm contracts.

In the relaxed position, the diaphragm is a dome-like structure. When it contracts it pulls the center down, thereby flattening itself. When it is flattened, the diaphragm increases the volume of the thorax, thereby decreasing air pressure inside the lungs, producing a vacuum. Air moves into the lungs from the higher pressure outside the body. When the diaphragm relaxes, the center of the diaphragm then moves back up into the thorax and thus decreases the volume in the thorax. The air is then pushed out, via the natural elastic recoil action of the lungs, diaphragm and chest wall.

Inhalation is the active part of breathing. Exhalation occurs passively, requiring no muscular effort under normal, restful circumstances. Chronic muscle tension in the thorax and/or involuntary muscle activity during exhalation prevents the normal rhythm of inhalation and exhalation. Lungs may not fill as deeply and evenly as they could; air may be pushed out by muscular effort rather than allowed to flow out. Sometimes controlling the air flow is desirable, as in speaking or singing. But as an unconscious habit pattern, excess muscle tension and activity reduce the options to change our breathing as our needs for oxygen, movement and expression change.

This pattern of breathing is like a signature and becomes a statement of one's way of being in the world. Thus, a Rosen worker looks to the breath for information. She wants to know the breathing pattern in order to work with the body, hoping to facilitate more options.

The diaphragm divides the thoracic cavity from the abdominal cavity. Passing through the diaphragm is the aorta, the main arterial blood vessel with blood leaving the heart; the inferior vena cava, the major vein coming from the lower extremities; and the esophagus. Due to their proximity, tension in the diaphragm is registered in these circulatory and digestive structures. Directly above the diaphragm, centrally positioned, is the heart and on either side of the heart are the lungs. Below the diaphragm on the left side are the stomach and the spleen and on the right side is the liver.

The action of the diaphragm is in direct contact with these organs due to fascial connections, thereby providing continuous passive involvement of them. When the diaphragm and the surrounding viscera have enough room to move, this lulling movement is believed in the Rosen scheme to contribute to these organs' wellness, by providing, in effect, an ongoing internal massage.

The diaphragm is innervated not only by the motor cortex of the brain, but also by a portion of the brain stem, which controls breathing at an autonomic level. During sleep or unconscious activity, this involuntary part of the brain regulates the contract/relax cycle of the diaphragm. The motor cortex is the voluntary part of the brain that allows one to breathe just as one desires, whether to speak, sing, or to do breathing exercises. Both voluntary and involuntary neurological input influence the diaphragm's action. Every muscle in the body will have a certain amount of voluntary and involuntary influence from the brain. But the diaphragm demonstrates its conscious and unconscious controls through its innervation by both nervous systems.

The diaphragm contracts, drawing air into the lungs, expanding the chest and passively moving the surrounding joints. The amount of oxygen made available to the body is determined by the depth and frequency of the diaphragm's action and the chest's ability to expand. The diaphragm's behavior is thus influenced by many parts of the brain that perceive and interpret the body's needs. Sensory detectors in the joints and muscles notify the brain to orchestrate the diaphragm to bring in more oxygen when they are stimulated by increasing physical activity or exercise. On the other hand, when at rest, the state of the somatic sensory endings support the brain's control of the diaphragm's slower, steadier breathing cycle, since less oxygen is required.

All psychological states and emotional responses have, as part of their experiential matrix, a physical expression, including a breathing pattern. For example, the diaphragm functions differently when one is quietly satisfied than when one is ecstatic. With a diaphragm that is not limited by intrinsic and/or extrinsic muscle tension, full emotional awareness and expression are available.

Resistance to emotional experience requires sequestering the physical sensations and actions that accompany such experience, generally by muscle tension and, more specifically, diaphragmatic tension. The breathing cycle reflects the repression via diminished movement of the diaphragm, chest and surrounding joint structures. As muscles relax and the breathing changes (i.e., increased movement and expansion of the chest), psychological and emotional shifts occur and support a greater sense of self-awareness.

Circulatory function is influenced by habitual, chronic muscle tension. When a region of the body is held rigid by tense muscles, blood flow into that region is restricted. As the muscles relax, more room is created around the blood vessels and blood can flow more easily into the surrounding tissues.

Some parts of the arterial system have muscle fibers in the walls of the vessels that assist the blood flow by contracting and relaxing. Veins have no muscle fibers in their connective tissue walls. Blood flow through the veins depends mainly on the contraction and relaxation action of surrounding muscles. When an area is held tight, blood does not circulate as freely as possible, denying the area full oxygenation, warmth and coloration.

The restricted blood flow also results in inefficient cellular waste removal from the muscle with resultant fatigue and pain. Moreover, tightened muscles trap fluids that begin to solidify and harden when kept static. Improved circulation aids in metabolizing such cellular waste products (e.g., lactic acid) via delivery of oxygen to the cell, then removes the remaining waste so that it can be expelled from the body.

Often, but not always, when blood circulation is improved and movement is reintroduced to a once-held part of the body, the sensory nerve endings are stimulated. This shift in physiological state may be experienced as uncomfortable, possibly painful. The Rosen worker maintains the awareness of the area, continues moving it and touching it. As the improved circulation and movement continue in the area, the soft tissue structures and joints physiologically adapt and the discomfort generally recedes. In some cases, the aching in the muscles may last for days, especially if long-held tension has been released. This aching pain is normal. However, a sharp or continual pain is sometimes a signal of injury and may be referred to a medical professional.

Skeletal Joints

The predominant type of joint in the body is the synovial joint. This type of bony junction is formed by two opposing surfaces covered by hyaline cartilage and surrounded by a fibrous joint capsule. Lining the capsule is the synovial membrane, which secretes and absorbs synovial fluid, the viscous lubricant of the joint. This fluid occupies the joint space between the bones. Movement of the joint stimulates production-reabsorption of the fluid, thereby nourishing and lubricating the articular cartilage.

When a joint is immobilized, less fluid is produced, the cartilage is not as nourished and lubricated as it should be and the connective tissues surrounding the joint begin to adhere. Movement is diminished and the condition may become painful in time if allowed to remain unconscious.

A Rosen worker looks for subtle passive movement in the joints of the body as the client breathes. A lack of movement indicates stiffness in and around the joint. The surrounding tense musculature may pull the bones closer together, thus decreasing the amount of synovial space between them. As muscles relax, the space increases, thereby allowing more movement and increasing production of synovial fluid.

Rosen Method addresses those areas that should move and yet do not move. With change, the body becomes more mobile and provides the options for movement that support the health of the joints, the muscles and the circulatory system. In Rosen Method, the degree of mobility and health within these systems serves as a metaphor for personal and philosophical ways of being in the world. The body tells the story. It is, in fact, a living autobiography.

4

TENSION AND HOLDING

Every muscular rigidity contains the history and the meaning of its origin. Its dissolution not only liberates energy . . . but also brings back into memory the very infantile situation in which the repression had taken place.

—Wilhelm Reich

The body tells the clearest what we want to hide the most.

—Marion Rosen

Rosen Method practitioners are in agreement with the basic premise of all bodywork: that without exception each body displays evidence of the body/mind connection. They see this connection as the foundation of their work.

The Puzzle of Limited Functioning

In scientific, descriptive terms, full body functioning is rare in adults. Rosen practitioners notice limited function through their knowledge of full movement, flexibility, agility and strength, believing that the reasons for diminished movement frequently lie in unconscious holding patterns. Those with material limitations such as broken bones, torn ligaments, sprains and strains, are not being discussed here. People presenting with such problems are referred to medical practitioners, although an emotional component in these cases is also acknowledged. Often the Rosen practitioner and the medical care provider work together.

To Rosen practitioners, psychosomatic clients are not seen as a group separate from the general population. We are all, in the Rosen scheme, psychosomatics, inasmuch as mind and body are inextricably linked.

Rosen theory evolved from physical therapy. Hospital workers have long known that patients who demonstrate a desire to regain normal health respond more readily to treatment. Because physical therapy attracts patients whose medical problems are often the result of physical trauma, the physical therapist observes closely a client's active participation in the healing process. The therapist's work involves the use of the hands as well: touching, gently probing and stretching. As a physical therapist, Marion Rosen began talking with patients about their injuries and their lives.

Thus, she shared intimately in her patient's healing. She found that patients who no longer had diagnosable disorders often continued to complain of pain, even though the supposed source of malfunction had ceased or healed. This group of patients puzzled Marion.

Another group of patients who also puzzled Marion seemed prepared to accept full bodily function, yet they made slow progress. In working with individuals of this type, Marion often used a direct, matter-of-fact approach.

> I was asked to see a man who was still limping more than three years after breaking his ankle. I had him walk around the room for a few moments while I carefully watched his body and feet. I could see no reason for the limp. When I asked him if he had to walk that way, he said, "No."
>
> I asked him to show me if he could walk without limping. He tried and walked normally. I asked him if it hurt to walk that way. He said, "No." I told him to continue walking that way then. He had forgotten how to walk, that was all.

Patients who had relatively minor body discomfort continued to make up a large segment of Marion's practice. They were the ones whose problems so fascinated Marion that her work with them led to the development of her theory and method. She recalls:

> I got interested in trying to see if it was somehow important for these patients to have their chronic pain. Pain is a guide if you let it be—a guide to tell us something is wrong and to do something about it. To have pain and let ourselves be in pain is a cry for help by the body. As I worked with my patients I started talking a little bit. I taught them movement. Sometimes they could do the movement and sometimes they couldn't. I also noticed that very often, as I loosened up some part of their bodies, they would start to talk. After a while I noticed that the people who talked seemed to get better the moment that they started to talk. The talk was what was really behind the work. Then I knew that in order for people to get better, they would have to talk.

Marion is quick to deny that she engaged in amateur psychological counseling:

In Marion's words:

> I talked to my patients but not as a therapist. I just talked with them. I was amazed to see how few people had anyone they felt free to talk with, even to the people closest to them. They would say things to me that they wouldn't say to anyone else—they would tell me so. I would wonder, why are they talking to me then? I saw a woman who said she had a wonderful life—a husband, children, money, everything—including a headache that wouldn't go away.
>
> Eventually in our conversations she complained that she never got to do what she wanted to do. When I asked her what that was, she said she wanted to sew. It seemed almost silly to me, because she was a woman who could afford to have all her clothes made, who certainly didn't have to sew. From the tone of her voice and the feeling I could sense moving through her body, I knew sewing was somehow important to her. I suggested she rearrange her schedule in order to give herself at least one hour a day to sew. I never saw her again. I learned years later that she never had headaches and she was still sewing. Patients with stories like hers allowed me to see that it is very important in life to let your creativity be active. Such a seemingly small self-denial had given her so much tension that she always had a headache.

But Marion's patients' symptoms weren't always relieved by simple suggestion. Many demonstrated creative adaptation to situations in their lives and, at least consciously, appeared to react and respond appropriately. Still, each suffered some measure of physical discomfort which was difficult to account for in medical terms. Many had been told by their doctors that they would have to "accept" their pain, to "learn to live with it."

What could be the cause of so much chronic pain and dysfunction? The reasons for lower back pain seemed to be almost as numerous as the individuals who suffered it. Certain gestures, specific postures, seemed to suggest general patterns, but they did not reveal a cause and effect relationship.

> I say that pain is a guide to tell us where we do something that is not good for our body. Pain is the body's cry for help. You are doing something that the body can't take any longer. The body is very patient; it takes a lot of tension and abuse before it makes pain.

Lessons from Dancers and Children in Movement

Marion Rosen remembered her observations of dancers during her stay in Sweden. Choreography is an attempt to make a language of body movement. Dance was exciting to Marion because of its ability to communicate ideas without verbalization. In dance, body movements interpret basic human emotions. Movements suggest supplication, thanksgiving, joy, withdrawal, expansiveness, nurturing and so on. Marion discerned in her patients an ability to express similar human emotions in a bodily way.

In developing her theory, Marion compared dance and language as communication forms. She saw them as complementary means of communication. Language, for which Marion possessed a singular talent, was the realm of description and logic. Dance, for which Marion possessed a strong sensitivity, was the realm of emotion and expressiveness. She watched her daughter and her daughter's playmates engage in children's fantasies, acting them out in combinations of language and movement. As a mother, she knew that a child's ability to demonstrate emotions was boundless.

Marion began to draw parallels between her observations of patients and of non-patient children. She took particular notice of phrases relating to the body as they were used in child rearing. Each time she heard an expression directing a child to use its body in a specific manner, she became interested: "don't touch," "stop yelling," "sit still," "no jumping," "don't cry." It became clear that the process of socialization contained abundant material to inhibit free, instinctual expression by the body. As she sensitized herself to such language, Marion discovered that the language was also replete with trite aphorisms for adult living founded on metaphors of the body: "keep a stiff upper lip," "don't lose your head," "brace yourself," "keep your chin up," "carrying the weight of the world on your shoulders," "tight ass," "brow beating," and many more.

The common thread between children and adults was the suppression of feeling and emotion. If a child expressed an emotion that was considered by an adult to be inappropriate, the child was criticized. Constant criticism of the emotive pattern modified the behavior, but the feelings which gave rise to the behavior were not expressed. Just at the time when a child was beginning consciously to experience emotions and feelings, the child was under pressure to stifle them.

Marion observed that the subjugation or suppression of emotions took place in a relatively short time frame, generally between the ages of two and six years. During that time, children learned to control their emotions with remarkable expediency, gaining short-term rewards for adopting the adult mode of suppressing bodily expression. Those who did not learn were labeled "problem children."

Marion's theory of child development comes from her work with adults. She noticed over the years that certain attitudes were expressed in the body and that these were based on events in the client's early childhood and in the socialization process itself. Her theory may be summarized as follows: The infant is totally dependent on the mother or some other adult for its growth and survival outside the womb. Continuous, ongoing acceptance and emotional commitment are essential on the part of the nurturing person to assure the infant's physical survival and emotional well-being.

The newborn human infant reacts in a completely instinctual manner to its new environment. The infant expresses its needs without inhibition. The nature of growth is revealed in children who, when not imposed upon, live in a state of constant exploration. Their seemingly insatiable curiosity and fascination reveals a strong desire to do and discover things by themselves. When not imposed upon, children know when, how much and what to eat; when to sleep; and when to wake up. They accept all parts and functions of themselves without making judgments that some are good or bad or dirty. They explore their environment and make their own evaluations about what is pleasant, desirable and satisfying. They trust their senses and are at ease with themselves and their discoveries.

Parents and other adults begin to influence the child's attitudes by exaggerating reactions and movements, talking baby talk, instructing the child in how to respond; say "hi," wave bye-bye, smile, say "please" and "thank you." A child loses his sense of self and no longer trusts that he knows what he wants or that his response is an expression of his own experience. In addition to normal language development, which occurs through participating fully in an ever-widening worldview, parents and other adults tend to impose abstract vocabulary that has no connection to the child's experience in an effort to hasten socialization.

If their play is interrupted to meet schedules, or their sleep is interrupted for the sake of convenience, children learn that there is no natural rhythm to life and that cutting things off in mid-stream is the way the world functions. In this process they lose their own internal rhythm and sense of self as being in harmony with the environment.

Thus begins the process of holding back, doubting, asking, deciding, "What should I be doing?" in response to any situation rather than expressing "How am I right now with what is happening?" Barriers between their own perceptions and expression of themselves have begun to develop and a film or veil forms between them and reality.

Typically children are not left to grow and develop according to their own feeling and inner guidance. Rather, outside influences play a major role in conditioning the child in expected preset ways. Thus the child comes to act and believe in ways which may be counter to his or her true and natural inclinations. If children are listened to and allowed freedom of expression in their play, they can later participate in activities, such as sports and dance, that encourage emotional expression through movement.

Socialization, however, is an inevitable process that has certain unfortunate by-products. As children grow, they learn to mute the signals their bodies send to their minds. Physical constriction in the body, as evidenced by tightening of the musculature, rigid posture and shallow breathing are the results of emotional constriction. Such tension is referred to as a barrier or holding.

Inhibition Becomes Body Tension

After her observation of children, Marion theorized that the energy that could have been used by the body to express emotions was being used instead to hold the emotions down. In her adult patients, Marion could see and feel muscular tension. She could relate it to her patients' stories of events in their lives. She hypothesized that their muscles were held in chronic tension as a reflection of inhibition against expressing certain feelings. The tension was consciously created in the beginning to hold back the impulse that could evoke an unwanted response from the adult in charge.

Over time the tension became chronic and patients were no longer aware of it. They were not letting themselves *be*; they had learned to *do* and not *be*. They were suppressing their emotions at the expense of their bodies. When working with her adult patients, Marion found that the longest-lasting barriers seemed to result from the loss of a parent through death or separation and/or a family move to a different home. Barriers resulted when the family was so preoccupied with the activity surrounding these events that the child was not listened to and his/her feelings were neglected.

According to Marion, the source of chronic tension is that the emotional experience has never found true expression. Muscle tension holds *down*, holds *in*, holds *together* emotions which may surface upon the release of the tension. Muscle tension is required to keep emotions under control, often to such a degree that one loses contact with what one is controlling.

As a physical therapist Marion had training and years of experience in seeing the effects of tension on the body. Now, discovery of the unconscious source of the tension implied that she would be dealing with her patients' unconscious material as she worked with their bodies.

In Marions words:

> What is in your body is in your unconscious. If you think you know what it is, that isn't what it is. The holding is an unconscious holding. You cannot tell that story. The story you can tell is made up of what you have already handled.
>
> Pain is a guide to the surfacing of what's unconscious, something repressed. The real pattern is in your unconscious and it hasn't surfaced yet. When it surfaces, it often takes care of the pain. Very often the pain disappears in the course of handling whatever the emotion was.
>
> It was very obvious that the area where the holding was, where there was stiffness or pain, the breath would not move. In the areas where they felt good, the breath would go back and forth. Very often as I worked on them, as they loosened up, the pain would go away just by virtue of the breath going to the spot. When that happened the pain would not come back over a long time.

How Breathing Relates to Tension

Marion had never relinquished the conviction, formed during her apprenticeship with Lucy Heyer, that breathing, while incompletely understood, was important in evaluation and treatment. She dealt with the obvious misuses of voluntary breathing patterns in her everyday practice. She was familiar with the patient who held his breath while trying to do the prescribed rehabilitation movements with a traumatized body area. Other patients hyperventilated when challenged by their own pain. She helped patients with either type of reactive breathing to resume a more natural breathing pattern. She taught her patients not to control their breathing in order to ease their pain and taught them that they could tolerate pain more readily if they overcame the tendency to control breathing. Patients who were less successful in allowing relaxed breathing to occur were, by Marion's estimation, also slower to heal.

Why did people change their breathing in an effort to control their pain, since unbeknownst to them it actually worked against that purpose? Marion began to discern a subtle correlation between limited breath and the patient's generalized body tension. The greater the breath in a natural, deep, relaxed way, the less tension there was. She postulated that a balance between muscular tension and easy, natural flow of breath could be achieved and would promote wellness.

Her interest in breathing grew when she compared the mechanisms of the musculature and the breath. The muscular action was voluntary, although conditioned unconsciously. Breathing was both involuntary and voluntary and framed by a conscious and unconscious process. The dual structure of the two systems, breathing and movement, seemed to suggest a double intersection.

She began to look for evidence to support her thesis. Marion was not a medical researcher. She was a superb clinician and she sought her empirical evidence with her senses sharply tuned to her patients. She noticed that the natural flow of breath in her patients' bodies correlated to the muscular tension that was present. With practice she discovered that much could be learned from observation, touch and verbal communication.

Marion continued to develop her skill as a "reader" of bodies. Her observations reinforced her discovery that the relaxation of muscle tension is the path to the unconscious, as the muscles hold the story of repressed emotions. She became absorbed in seeking information to alleviate patients' discomforts via a total body assessment. Objective questioning revealed only what was conscious; assessment of the body revealed the unconscious as well. She found that the unconscious material being contacted by her hands, along with her words, could often come into awareness and be expressed by the client, not out of the cognitive brain, but from the felt emotional sources in the body.

Marion has never lost her focus as a physical therapist. She wants to facilitate the relaxation of tension; unexpressed emotion is the source of tension. It is not always necessary to address the unconscious material that causes the repression of emotion because the body provides, through both the breath and the musculature, its own barometer of change. Marion disregards verbal material if it is not accompanied by bodily expression. While she sees the mind and body as interconnected, her focus is the body.

If a client's tension or holding seems to be rooted more deeply in the psyche than in the musculature, Marion or the practitioner refers him to an appropriate specialist. If the client responds in his body, the session can go forward with the confidence that the client has the ability to integrate the unconscious material into his overall experience.

> What we are working with is the tension in people's bodies, the holdings. What I mean by that is a muscle that is contracted and has forgotten to release. A muscle can do two things. A muscle can contract and a muscle can release. That's all a muscle can do—work and not work. Strength is the potential between relaxing and contracting. A muscle that is already contracting to hold back cannot do anything else. If you want to be strong, you have to start with muscles in the relaxed state.
>
> What makes strength is being vulnerable, being soft, being lackadaisical and then having the possibility to put the muscle through its range and have a full contraction. A normal body has that everywhere. When you look at a child, for instance, you find most everything moves at all times, totally. It freezes for maybe a second and then it goes immediately into movement again. This is how we were made.

Rosen Method turns patients' problems inside out. Clients are not people simply with psychogenic disorders; they are people who can be reached and guided toward maximum wellness through this work.

5

PROCESS

I was a prisoner carrying a heavy load of bones and flesh, but I have broken the chains of my muscle-bound body by the power of relaxation. I am free. Now I shall try to go within.

—Paramahansa Yogananda

When you touch clients in a way that frees them, that makes them feel acknowledged, there is a wave that goes through the body. Sometimes all that is necessary is for them to be listened to, to be looked at and touched. It's a great thing and well worth the time you put in with the person.

—Marion Rosen

The mind-body relationship is intricate. The Rosen worker does not know what the client knows. She knows when the client has connected with his unconscious by noticing the relaxation of tense areas and the free movement of the breath. The practitioner is able to see only physical changes in the client.

Other indications that the client has connected with unconscious material are fluttering of the eyelids, changes in facial expression, agitation, stomach gurgles, swallowing, tearing of the eyes, or twitching.

Many experiences relate to pre-verbal origins. Some clients report experiences that they believe relate to pre-natal origins. The practitioner can see only what is happening outside the body; she must word questions to evoke a response from the body and not particularly invite a verbal answer. The practitioner must avoid drawing conclusions about the client's internal state and must limit her observations to changes that can be seen or felt. Often the changes are so subtle they are easy to overlook. However, many small changes over time can result in a more fully embodied sense of self and are just as important as the dramatic changes that sometimes occur. There is no value judgment placed on how connections and changes are made.

> That's the reason I think this work, in the physical realm, is slower; because we do not impose. It's always the route toward something. You do not know who the person is and they don't know either. That is the premise of the work. They really do not know or have forgotten who they are . . .
>
> If I say in a few words where we want to go with the work, it is just getting to know our inner reality, getting in touch with who you really are, getting also in touch with what you put out there, what you play at being. As you slowly allow this and become aware of how you play and let go of some of the role playing you find that there is something beyond that, that is really you.

Rosen Method is not a mechanical process. It is a journey taken together by client and practitioner toward self-discovery. The process and technique can best be described by tracing the events of a hypothetical session.

The Beginning of the Session

The session begins when the client enters the room. The practitioner starts by making close but seemingly casual observations of the client's state of being. The practitioner begins to gather information from the client's movements, body attitudes and voice. The practitioner is interested in forming a sense of how the client presents and expresses himself.

> The way we get in touch with the client's emotions in the search for the real person is to get the clues in the body. First, in the picture that the person presents with their body; second, in the muscular tension we can feel in their body; and third, which is the most definite, how a person allows their breath to move through the body.

A first session usually begins with a few questions. The practitioner may ask, "How did you come to make an appointment?" or "What do you hope to get out of this session?" or, "What's going on in your life that makes you want Rosen Method now?" or, "What brings you here?" This initial questioning begins the collection of a brief but important history.

Practitioners are taught to recognize the limitations of this work—that it is not medical treatment—and to screen clients accordingly. Rosen Method is not appropriate for all potential clients. There are times in life when we have to hold ourselves together in order to survive: for example, after the loss of a loved one. Holding makes it possible to get through day to day life until gradually, over time, one can deal with the loss. Psychotic people often have a poor sense of boundaries and our work would not serve them. People who have pain that has not responded to medical treatment often need that pain for a variety of reasons unknown to both client and practitioner. The practitioner best serves this client by declining to work on him. Practitioners are cautioned to stay within the limits of their own discipline and expertise.

A client will be asked to remove what clothes he is comfortable removing. If the client is comfortable in just underpants, the work is a little easier. The areas not being worked on will be covered with a sheet.

The client lies on the table and makes himself comfortable. Clients are most often asked to lie face down because there are larger muscles to work with on the back and because they are likely to feel less vulnerable in this position with the belly and throat protected. A small, thin pillow is sometimes placed under the hips and another pillow is placed under the insteps or ankles to alleviate tension in the lower back and legs.

Exploring for Tension

The practitioner begins by looking at the back to see where the muscles appear to be tense, where the breath moves freely and where it is withheld, thereby getting a general idea of the statement the client makes with his body. For example, does he take up as much space as he is meant to occupy? What is the direction of the holding? Does he bear down on himself, hold himself together, puff himself up or separate his top from his bottom by tightening around his middle?

These questions are asked silently and the observing and evaluation done quickly so that the client is not made to feel like a specimen.

The practitioner then runs her hands gently over the client's body, still gathering information and comparing what she has seen with what she is now feeling beneath her hands. The task is to expand slowly his awareness of himself and to invite relaxation. Once the client has "dropped in," she might begin talking with him about what she is observing. She must be non-judgmental and non-directive in speaking with the client. For example: "There is holding here, in your support area," rather than, "Your hips are too broad," or, "You are resisting."

While speaking to the client, the practitioner watches the body. Questions or statements are intended to bypass the thinking mind and evoke a response from the body. If the practitioner's words evoke a response, it will be expressed in the client's body. The movement of the breath will show in that area or quickly be held back; the tension in the muscles might soften, or a flush of color might come into the area.

The practitioner watches and feels for the place on the client's back that is most unmoving, held, or not included in his expression of himself. He is unaware of what he is holding back. As she works, she goes a little deeper with her touch to contact the muscles at their level of holding and she feels a slight "giving" in the tension. At this point, the client may have an awareness of what happened that made the holding necessary in the first place and a softening will occur. As the muscle softens and relaxes, she follows the response with her touch.

Often the practitioner sees the change before the client feels it in himself. She might notice that the contracted muscle smoothes out, the shape of the area changes and the movement of the breath can be seen. Sometimes it becomes apparent that he has allowed all of the opening or softening in his back that he can and that work on the front might now be more productive. She might then ask the client to turn over.

The action of the client's diaphragm is more visible when he lies on his back. Since the diaphragm is the major muscle involved in breathing, its action reveals whether or not there is still holding. It is easier to see the tension patterns from the front.

Sometimes as the practitioner works with the muscles that move with the diaphragm, a flutter of the diaphragm itself can be seen. Movements in the abdomen might begin as they do when a person is crying or sobbing, although the expression on the face has not changed, leading her to believe that the sadness that is being expressed in the body is not reaching the face and the consciousness of the client.

She then looks for the places around the neck and chest that he tightens in order to hold down the emotion felt in the lower body. As she works in that area, he starts to become aware of the sadness and an expression of sadness comes over the face. After a while a few tears might appear in the eyes and the sob that had been seen in the abdomen and diaphragm might then begin. Often the face takes on the look of the age at which that particular experience took place.

The practitioner might then ask what happened at the age she thinks the face is portraying. The practitioner sees and feels a change taking place in the body, brings the client's awareness to it with the movement of her hands and asks him a question or makes a statement about the process and her observations. The client's awareness comes into that place and the emotional content of the experience that had been withheld becomes conscious.

> As all tension contains emotions that have been repressed, this is the direct route to contact the emotions. The work consists of a massage designed to relax the musculature. It is actually more specific than massage. It is working directly with the area that is holding and staying with it long enough to have something happen. Then the words we use are there to bring awareness to the changes that take place in the body through relaxation and will also acknowledge some emotions that are being made visible by not holding back. Not holding back is relaxation. Then the emotions that have been repressed can surface.

Marion offers two examples from a classroom demonstration:

> **Case 1:** I worked on a psychiatrist in his late forties who had undergone seven years of analysis. I noticed that there was a lot of tension around his diaphragm that made his stomach stick out even as he was lying on his back. As I worked around his diaphragm, I told him that this is where we hold when we feel anxious. This is the way the body represses anxiety. He said he had been anxious all his life. As I kept working, his breathing changed and his facial expression became that of a seven year old. I asked him what happened when he was seven.
>
> He gave a deep sob and began to talk. His father, whom he loved dearly, had died at that age. He was the eldest of

three children. Before he died, his father had told him, "You will have to help your mother now. You are the man in the family." He recalled the fear that swept through him and he recalled thinking, "How can I? I'm so little." That was the essence of his experience.

I did not work any further at that time, as I felt that contact with one deep experience is all I want out of one session. The ramifications of it continue to work on in the person afterward. After he got up and was dressed he told me he had spent seven years of his analysis on that incident, but he had never experienced what it had actually felt like. And the relief to him was indescribable. But he was also interested to notice that his stomach didn't protrude anymore, as the diaphragm had started its normal swinging function.

Case 2: I worked on a middle-aged woman during a demonstration. As the tight musculature between her shoulder blades was touched, she began trembling. Her expression quickly changed from sad to glad to surprise and she finally took on the look of a puzzled child around the age of six. When I asked her what happened when she was six or seven years old, she told of being a child in London during the bombing. She told of being evacuated from the city with other children and going to live with relatives in the countryside.

Her father was in the army and her mother remained in London where she was killed by a bomb. There was no emotion or "truth" in the body as this story was told. When I asked, "What else?" tears filled the woman's eyes. She told of her father's visits, describing him as dashing, debonair and full of fun. He would sweep her into his arms, dance around the room with her and make her laugh. She loved him dearly and was completely taken by him. Soon, though, he would go away leaving her feeling destitute and alone. He popped in and out of her life in this way for many years before he died.

In the session she realized that it was her father she had yearned for all her life. The loss of her mother had somehow been accepted and integrated by the child but not the loss of her father.

She could later reflect on the effect the loss of her father had on her life and relationships. The bombing, evacuation, life in the country, mother's death and visits by her father were familiar. She had told of them many times. But the felt experience of herself as a small child, wanting her father to stay with her, was new. As she felt it, her back softened, allowing the muscles that had been held to be available for reaching out to make contact with others.

What Client and Practitioner Experience

Each session is a fresh experience for both practitioner and client. There may be no apparent continuity through a series of sessions. Progress is not always traceable. The practitioner approaches each session from an "unknowing," as she has not shared this particular moment with this client before. The practitioner learns to become comfortable with ambiguity and non-attachment to results. She can never predict what will happen or even be sure that something will happen. Clients accept the fact that they have embarked on a journey toward self-discovery and that what surfaces each time is more of themselves.

The practitioner works with the chronic muscular tension needed to maintain a posture that masks the client's authentic self. When the early experience that required the posture and subsequent holding is re-experienced and the feelings associated with it are expressed, one can change one's position or way of standing or moving. The practitioner is there to bring the client's attention to the holding. Often it appears that not much has happened during a session, but when the client comes in for the next session he may share that memories, feelings and long-forgotten incidents have come into his awareness since his last visit. Sometimes this re-emergence of material from the past is unsettling for the client and he might need reassurance that it is an expected part of Rosen Method.

The constant effort required to produce and maintain an unnatural posture requires much energy. When an unnatural posture is maintained over a period of time, it becomes unconscious. It is seen then as a condition of chronic tension or holding in the body. When this tension lets go, the energy that was needed for holding becomes available for living. Clients often report feeling energetic or lighter.

> All we want is for a person to get connected with what they're holding back. The degree to which they repress, that they will not allow themselves to experience; that they carry around with them. All these things we carry around within ourselves actually interfere and form a barrier to our living. They are like loads, like rocks in our being.

When practitioners look at bodies they note the function of whatever muscles are held and direct their questions to help the client understand that his holding impedes the natural function of the muscles. For example, the muscles around the shoulder blades and along the outside of the ribs move the arms. The arms reach out to interact with others, to give as well as to receive and to express creativity. When these muscles are held down or in or together, the client is restraining himself from free expression with his arms.

There is no chart or map of the body used in Rosen Method. The practitioner is seeing and feeling the limitations to natural function that the client has placed on himself. The questions asked by the practitioner are meant to bypass the thinking mind and evoke a response from the body. Such questions or statements do not always require or elicit a verbal response. The purpose of the questioning is for the client to uncover the underlying need for his holding. Students and practitioners learn to trust the process of each session, being careful not to project their own meaning upon a client's experience. Tension in the leg muscles might suggest the individual has "taken a firm stand," feels it necessary "to stand and take it," is not ready "to step out," or other symbols of their repressed emotions and actions.

> **Case 3:** A client in her forties came for treatment for several months. Her legs were tight and as they were worked on she remembered that when she was a youngster she wanted to run away from home. She had to hold herself back from doing so because she knew she couldn't survive on her own. As the tension in her legs let go, she felt a sense of freedom and of readiness to move ahead in her life. She was surprised though and nearly overwhelmed by the return of her sexual feelings that had been suppressed by the holding in her legs.

In this case, held-in sexuality was not bringing about the tension. Rather, the repression of feelings, carried as tension, was interfering with sexuality. Sexual dysfunction was not the problem; it was a by-product of the holding.

The practitioner may or may not verbalize impressions to the client. There are no predictable guidelines for the student or practitioner. An ability to know precisely when to speak and when not to is part of the reason for training by apprenticeship. Marion instructs her trainees as follows:

> The way to find the strength and the possibilities for movement in your clients is to give up what you are holding on to, what you are certain about. You have to have a strong commitment to going through that place in yourselves. It will happen every time you start working on somebody. You go through this phase of who am I and what am I going to do? And from that comes your strength every time. You are not certain. You are never certain. So every time you work you are sure nothing will happen. You have to go through that in order to really connect with your knowledge, with your being (essence) and with your strength. It will happen every time. But know that

it is part of your possibility to move ahead. Your possibility to perceive what is going on with the client. And what comes then is really a knowledge that is in you. As you work more and more you get in touch with your knowledge.

Practitioners learn through their training to use words and touch to bring awareness to the client of his bodily response. The practitioner is a body reader, not a mind reader.

The End of the Session

A session lasts about an hour. As it draws to a close, the practitioner lets the client know by saying, "I am going to stop in a few minutes," implying that the client's unfolding will continue even after the session, or she will simply say, "I'm going to stop now."

At the end of a session, the practitioner stops working and pulls the sheet up to cover the client. The client is encouraged to stay on the table and rest for a few minutes before getting up and dressing. The practitioner might make a mental note for her own interest of how the client's appearance compares with her initial impressions. She might notice that there is more movement of the breath through the body, softness in the face, clarity in the eyes, or resonance in the voice. It is, however, impossible to evaluate the full effect of a session accurately at the end of a session. The effects of the client's simply letting go continue after the session.

If the client needs more time to rest, he may be invited to sit in the waiting room and perhaps have a cup of tea or take a walk before driving away; thus allowing the client time to integrate the experience that he had on the table and to redirect his attention to the outer world before moving on.

Often, after a private session or classroom demonstration, a client will say that he doesn't feel different at all, or that although he feels relaxed, nothing really happened. One such client returned the next week and sheepishly reported that on the way home he drove into a ditch. Another reported pulling into a gas station and bursting into tears as he rolled down the window when the attendant approached. It is a good idea, then, to advise the client to leave some free time after a session.

Sometimes the practitioner can see and feel that the client has made a connection between the tension in his body and an unconscious event. When she asks the client what happened, the client might report that there is nothing there, no images, thoughts, or emotions—just a feeling of more space within himself. Such a feeling might be connected to a pre-verbal experience. Some clients have even connected feelings to events that took place before they were born, which they were later able to verify with the help of a parent or sibling.

Often there is just a gradual softening of the tight musculature as the client gains a more complete experience of himself and reduces the area he has to hold back. He accepts himself more fully as he is, with less watching, less caution and less restriction. It is not always important to know what has been released.

Marion offers a case to illustrate this point:

Case 4: A young woman came for a session in a state of total exhaustion. She hadn't been able to work. I saw her regularly for a long time. Nothing happened except that she got just a little more relaxed. No big insights, no big changes. She just got progressively more energetic, had more joy in living and was more in touch with her own power. After a while, we had to agree that she was a very high-powered, healthy and successful person in her private and professional life. And neither of us knew what happened. Over time, the state of her tension changed. The quality of her breathing changed. The barriers never made themselves known. Whatever was there just disappeared. She came for sessions for over two years and continued for many more months after agreeing that she had made important changes.

Sometimes people are helped by simply getting in touch with the enormous amount of physical tension they have or with how they have allowed the demands of their life to encroach on their feelings.

Rosen Method sessions provide an opportunity for the client to unveil the feeling behind the holding, not by dissection but by finding the emotion in the body so that it can be recognized. Each session is intended to stimulate something, to teach something. Clients go their own way; the way they are going is toward becoming themselves and making more space for *being* rather than *doing*. That feeling is one of well-being.

6

WHEN EMOTIONS SURFACE

Rigidity functions as a defense as long as the rigidity is unconscious, that is, as long as the person is unaware of his rigidity or its meaning.
                                                    —Alexander Lowen, M.D.

Many of the events are not important. It is what that event means to the person at the time that is important. These feelings are held tightly in the body and then overlaid by a very nice stance the person has taken to cover it all up. The holding is still there on the inside and that holding forms a barrier against movement, function and interaction with the outside world. This makes a very deep and constant repression.
                                                    —Marion Rosen

In Marion's words, "It's not the big upheaval things that very often count. It's the little things that all of a sudden we see as the key to some way we have directed our lives."

Opening New Bodily Possibilities

Rosen Method can be compared metaphorically to the sculptor's task—chipping away at the holding musculature until the person underneath can emerge. Movement in the muscles brings the client's holding to his awareness. The client's body is a monument that he has built to himself.

Relaxation of tension in a held muscle is the tangible indication of change and brings potential for further release. The muscle that is now relaxed has the possibility of remaining relaxed, to contract again only as actually necessary for healthy function. If the muscle changes and the movement of the breath comes into the area, an emotional release has occurred. Emotional release and muscular release are interdependent—one does not occur without the other. This interdependence flows directly from the connection between mind and body.

The trigger for release is unconscious. Clients who experience the release of muscular tension in this way report an overall sense of well-being. Rosen Method practitioners attribute this sense to the release of repressed emotions whether or not the client became aware of them during the session. Often, repressed emotions become conscious later on, after the session has ended and the client is involved in something else.

This release of tension produces new possibilities for both the muscles and the emotions. The muscles regain their natural flexibility for movement. Marion Rosen defines strength as the potential of the muscle to go from shortened and held to lengthened and relaxed; in other words, from working to non-working.

The new possibility in the client's emotional life is to feel emotions as they arise. The experience of the release of repressed emotion teaches the client that repression is no longer necessary and the choice whether to express or suppress becomes a possibility. Many clients connect with the experience that caused the holding. The connection is a re-experiencing or reminder of the emotional content, often of a memory, from a perspective altered by time. The emotional release brings about an improved sense of well-being. Even in clients who do not connect to the experience that originally produced the repression, release is still felt in the form of relaxation.

When we work with people, often they start to cry and say, "I don't know why I'm crying, I have nothing to cry about." But the crying is coming. This is what I call pure emotions. At that point they cannot connect any pictures, any experiences. It is just that feeling of wanting and needing to cry.

The same thing happens about joy and laughter. Sometimes it just bubbles up without anything happening. People start laughing or giggling or start saying, "I feel so happy," and for some reason, that kind of emotion had been repressed.

It seems very strange to have an emotion like happiness or laughter be repressed. But in one instance, a man remembered when he was a young child at his father's funeral and the people were all in dark clothes and he started giggling because he thought it looked so funny, the people all with serious faces and acting strange. When he started giggling, his mother turned to him and told him he was a heartless, awful person to giggle at his father's funeral. He stopped laughing and he did not laugh anymore. And every time things were funny, he seemed to have repressed it all his life. He could not remember laughing.

And this is what came up in the treatment. All the repressed laughter, joy. And you could see how his life changed by allowing himself to use this emotion again or acknowledge it. But as it had come at first, it was just the pure emotion. After talking awhile, we got to the picture of what had happened—which he had forgotten.

Sometimes emotion emerges as pure emotion; there is no "story" that accompanies it. The client does not have a memory of a specific event in the past. The inability to connect the unconscious content of the client's experience to an historical event does not diminish the importance or effect of the release. The power of Rosen Method is that as muscles are relaxed the feeling is directly experienced. Other forms of therapy focus on events in clients' lives, trying to uncover how the client feels or felt about events. Rosen Method focuses on the muscular tension that holds the feelings in, allowing the events that produced them to be revealed, or not:

> You [the client] may think you know what it is. You think you had difficulties with your mother and then when the release comes, you find out it wasn't your mother at all. It was your father or a brother the real emotion got stuck on. And it was the real emotion that formed the barriers and that is what is in your body and that is what you can feel and we [practitioners] can feel with our hands and see.
>
> I say again and again, when we work on somebody we have no idea what is really going on with that person. We just have no idea. You absolutely cannot know anything when you start working on a person. And all you're doing is witnessing their coming out, their getting to know themselves. They are coming to life in a different way, as barriers they didn't know existed before are touched and allowed to disappear.
>
> The difficulty about these things is that they are unconscious, that they are really not known. They are not memories. They are emotions gone beyond the conscious and then all of a sudden without thought, without effort, it comes out. And the first thing is the emotion that was experienced.

What Happens When Emotions Surface

- Emotions sometimes come up as pure emotion, not connected to anything;

- Sometimes there are mental pictures from the past—of certain incidents or ways of living that could not be dealt with in childhood;
- The person is faced with the experience and has a chance to deal with it now as an adult when he or she could not deal with it when it happened;
- The moment the experience becomes conscious it does not need to be repressed anymore, so the cause of the tension is removed and the person can function in the area that up to now was unavailable;
- There are many more or less significant areas of suppression in most of us. In some of us it is so extensive that the body cannot function normally anymore;
- In some of us it has crippled us emotionally as our realm of action has been critically reduced.

By reversing these processes, we regain our former ability to function. In the end, we come to a point of choice, of wanting to face our emotions, to handle our lives, to fully live as human beings, or to stay in the confinement of our repressions. The choice in the end is ours, but the possibilities are there through this work.

Increasing Consciousness

In many types of therapy the goal is to bring into consciousness that which is unconscious. In Rosen Method, consciousness usually comes spontaneously with the surfacing of the emotion. The emotion, held by the muscles, is directly contacted and is not dependent upon finding the "story" that the client is keeping repressed. The muscular release brings the emotion into consciousness. The area of the body that has responded to touch and has released its tension has the possibility of regaining full functioning. The muscles remain functional as long as no new emotional holding is required.

By re-experiencing or remembering long-held emotions, it becomes possible to experience emotions spontaneously. If an emerging emotion is too difficult for the client to experience, the practitioner feels the bodily response of holding more tightly along with the restricted movement of the breath.

In Marion's words:

> Clients unconsciously contract the muscles in order to keep
> an emotion away. They cannot accept the emotion. If a client
> chooses not to feel, or they are still not able to handle the emo-
> tion, they can shut off and tighten against it.

Clients who release emotions feel relief and expansiveness. Most are
stunned by the simplicity of the experience. The client usually tells the
practitioner what has happened. The practitioner confirms the change
by noting the relaxation in the muscles and the movement of the breath
and by acknowledging the feelings of the client.

Rosen Method practitioners are trained to pay attention to the relationship between themselves and their clients. They seek to create an atmosphere conducive to intimacy but to avoid being caught up in the client's
emotions. Practitioners try to be present and acknowledge, validate and
support the experience for the client without taking it up or taking it on in
any way that would diminish it for the client. Rosen practitioners refer to
this delicate balance as both "being with" and "getting out of the way."

These special moments occur with frequency and may revolve around
large emotional events or around seemingly trivial occurrences. Because
they happen frequently, the practitioner has ample opportunity to gain
skills to handle the moment. With practice it becomes possible to be
present, get out of the way, and allow the client to have his own experience. The practitioner is the facilitator of the client's experience, not the
initiator of it.

> What I often do to avoid taking a client away from the expe-
> rience by talking about it is to say I would like to talk about
> it later. Maybe at the next session, to give them time to see
> for themselves what happened. More often than not they will
> know what they need to do with it. What we are doing is get-
> ting them in touch with the barriers they put there. With the
> parts of them that they have been hiding from themselves.

And allowing them to look at whatever they've been hiding, so as not to hold there anymore.

What they do with it then is a matter of choice. Sometimes they need therapists. Many of the people I work with have therapy at the same time. For us as Rosen practitioners, we get them in touch with what they didn't know about themselves, then they see if they can handle it. For instance, when they get in touch with how they hold people away, how every time there is any possibility of somebody getting close to them, how they shut off. And they get in touch with their degree of shutting off. Then they can say, "I know I'm doing it and maybe next time I can catch myself before I do it." With knowing this they can change things. When they don't know, they can't change it . . . they have no choice.

When a client re-experiences an event that, even from his adult standpoint, is difficult to handle, he may be referred to a psychotherapist. When something is experienced in one session, it does not mean that resolution has taken place. The client is now on his way to integrating that experience into his life. He is bound to the past only if the experience and feelings associated with it remain repressed. The practitioner remains present with her hands lightly on the client. This is the moment of that delicate balance where the practitioner can both "be there and keep out of the way."

The emotional release brings most clients instant information about themselves. Contrary to their expectation that their emotions would be too powerful or overwhelming, clients learn that they can survive their own emotions and become more open to their emotions as they arise.

For some, the release is an apocalyptic event; they feel as they have never felt before. For others, full acceptance and integration is a gradual process. But all are moved by re-experiencing the events they have long held repressed in their bodies. The naturalness of the emotional release and expression overrides the client's habitual way of holding.

Clients who re-experience emotion through Rosen Method do so directly; that is, they experience emotions spontaneously. They know what they are feeling. They experience their emotions and describe them either as pure feeling or through a personal story that, to them, explains the emotion. The body/mind responds immediately to the surfacing of long-held emotion. The experience has both short-term and long-term results. The muscles have changed and increased their potential for strength. The mind has increased its potential for expansion and consciousness has been awakened.

The goal of Rosen Method is to bring awareness to the possibilities that have been lost through holding, primarily in the body. The body/mind interdependence means that the mind and the body opens up to possibilities that did not exist before. The openings present an opportunity for the client to go beyond his present reality, perhaps to transcend common levels of consciousness and attain a sense of wholeness: "To thine own self be true."

Anger, Sadness, Fear and Love

Marion Rosen recognizes a hierarchy of primary emotions that can be ranked from the more accessible to the deepest: anger, sadness, fear and love. In Marion Rosen's words:

> When we get to our loving we are really vulnerable. But once you open up any repressed emotion, they all come up. You can't hold just one down and you can't just let one up. But it seems that sadness and anger are repressed at a higher level than fear. Fear, I feel, is more in the middle and the love seems to be way down. Love and relationships seem to be around the heart. But really deep, total loving seems to be much lower in the body, where the legs connect with the pelvis, where we allow ourselves to move and not to move. Essential fear and deepest love are found there; that is, the repression of it is found there. I can only say that when I work on people there and when that holding lets go, then the love comes through. Deep love, deep fear.

In her view, the repression of anger and sadness is often found in the neck and top of the torso. Feelings toward others are repressed around the heart and upper middle of the trunk. Relationships and love on a personal level are also felt there. Fear and anxiety are repressed around the diaphragm. Universal love, always the last emotion to surface, is felt deep in the belly. When that moves, people feel pure love, love that is not connected to anything or anyone—the love that *is*.

In Marion's view, anger, sadness and fear are easier to admit to in our culture than love. Anger is a response to somebody or something and is connected to hurt, loss, or frustration. She believes that guilt, embarrassment and confusion are secondary and are not expressed or released through the body; these feelings are expressed as stories.

Fear, also a primary emotion in the Rosen scheme, is felt in response to an event (either in the moment or in retrospect) and has a story connected to it. As with love, however, there is a much deeper experience of fear that is repressed deep in the bottom of the torso, where the legs and pelvis connect. This sort of fear seems to threaten one's very existence, one's very being and is very deeply and tightly held. When that fear lets go, the struggle is gone from one's life and the possibility of moving freely with life instead of holding against it becomes available.

> There are many areas in our body in which these things happen. In our legs, our backs, our shoulders. There are other things, too, like in our neck—we want to talk, we want to yell, we want to cry. There are muscles there that hold us back when we are told "don't cry," "little boys don't cry," "pull yourself together," "what have you got to cry about," "don't do that." And you start swallowing and not crying. And the next time you start to cry you remember someone said you shouldn't cry. You start holding back right away without being told.
>
> After a while, when you feel like crying, you immediately hold there. So the conscious act of "I have to hold back" is not there anymore and the jump over from the feeling to the holding has been made. You no longer have the feeling, just the repression of it, the stiff neck, the tight shoulders and chest.
>
> When we work on these areas and the muscles begin to

loosen, very often people start to cry. And there is nothing sad happening to them, but it seems as if there is a body memory of all the times they had to suppress crying.

No map or blueprint of the body is used to identify certain emotions as being repressed or held by specific muscles. The practitioner derives the correspondence between emotions and muscle groups from her common-sense understanding of muscle function. For example, if a person needs to suppress crying or yelling, he will tighten his neck and chest. If he needs to repress fear, he will tighten around his diaphragm. If he gives into resignation, he will collapse his chest. The practitioner considers muscle function when looking for clues as to what might be held in the body. The truth of the holding comes from the client in the form of bodily response to touch and words.

Rosen Method students are taught to notice the movement in the body that happens when emotions arise. They learn to be open to other people's feelings and to encourage them to communicate them.

Rosen Method is not cathartic work. During a session, emotions are not acted out. To act out emotions is to *do* them and doing them gets in the way of feeling them. When emotions are re-experienced through Rosen Method, they are sometimes experienced with a sigh. Expanded internal space fills with the movement of breath, often in just a few seconds. The insight gained in such moments sometimes needs a much longer time, days or weeks, in order to be processed and integrated.

An important learning for clients and students is in understanding the difference between "experiencing" and "doing" a feeling. People often believe that if they allow their anger, sadness, love or fear to come out, they will be overwhelmed by it or that they will have to do something about it. Rosen Method points out that feelings are simply feelings, not the events themselves and that the way to handle feelings is to experience them as they happen. Through this work the "doing" in the body / mind that inhibits the expression is contacted and the client may become aware of new possibilities.

7

ACCEPTANCE, SURRENDER,
SPIRITUALITY

We shall not cease from exploration
And the end of all our exploring
Will be to arrive where we started
And know the place for the first time   —T.S. Eliot

This work is about transformation—from the person we think we are to
the person we really are. In the end, we can't be anyone else.

—Marion Rosen

Through Rosen Method, old habits, attitudes and ways of being are contacted and brought to awareness by the relaxation of chronic tension in the body. Physical relaxation allows for more space in the body and in the mind. Into this space comes the possibility of new ways of expression that are more authentic to the true nature or essence of the person.

When the diaphragm relaxes and moves freely, self-acceptance and surrender have occurred. The diaphragm is incapable of relaxation through conscious effort. Surrender is allowing, not performing: Effort interferes with the process. The diaphragm is more fully involved in surrender than any other muscle; its release is a sign that deep emotions have been felt.

The free movement of the diaphragm is the indicator that contact has been made with the underlying unconscious attitude that has determined the client's world-view. Here is an example:

> **Case 5:** During a session a woman talked about the death of her mother. The woman was six at the time of the mother's death and had been stoic about the loss. As the old feelings about missing her mother were contacted, along with rigidity in her body, she began to cry and the feelings flooded in.
>
> It would seem that this incident should be the end of the session. However, since her diaphragm did not swing freely and the free movement of breath did not fill her chest, it was obvious that there was more to her story. By working with the tight place around her mid-section, I felt muscular rigidity along both sides of her spine. The client said that she had a mental image of a superstructure surrounding her spine. I asked, "What do you need the superstructure for?" The client replied that she felt she needed more support than her back could give her. When asked what she needed extra support for, she said, "To get ready for the next disaster." With that, her diaphragm released, her back relaxed and her breath moved in to fill her torso. Her life-stance was an unconscious statement: "I always have to be ready for the next disaster."

Before the session, the woman had rigid posture with her head thrust forward and her shoulders held high. After her back relaxed, her shoulders softened and dropped to a more natural position and her head and neck were in alignment with her spine. She realized then, as she talked about the session, that she had been using her head as a periscope, always alert for the next disaster.

When the client accepts and acknowledges himself, space opens up and new ways of expression become possible. The authentic self, or essence, is contacted and becomes available.

One's worldview is kept limited by chronic muscular tension. When the limitation is discovered and acknowledged, the tension required to maintain it lets go. The energy that was used for holding is then available for living. New possibilities for responding to events in one's life open up and the energy needed for a new worldview is available. This experience can be both humbling and exhilarating. The client realizes he has not been wrong, only that he has been limited, as if he had been seeing with blinders on. He has not acquired more knowledge, but a new knowing; a shift in consciousness.

Consciousness may be the most powerful force in the universe and the body, and with its senses and its nervous system, may be the vehicle through which that power manifests. When consciousness flows into the world through a felt sense of the body/mind connection, change is no longer threatening and successive layers of self-discovery follow on one another.

In Rosen Method, entry to the transformation process is made through the body, which then becomes the map of this new territory. The body tells the truth about one's inner reality.

The client has a new view of himself and may have difficulty integrating parts of his old life into his new way of living. He may no longer enjoy the same pastimes, friends, or work. He may feel out of place. He cannot go back and he may not know how to go forward. He may at this time need more traditional psychotherapeutic help with the integration process. He may simply need time alone to understand and assimilate the new experience. He may explore new interests, new relationships and new possibilities in an attempt to validate his experience of himself.

As the process of self-discovery unfolds, the client becomes aware of the many levels of holding in his body and of how the withholding has impacted his life. In Marion's view, the emotion that clients hold back the most is their love. When they feel their own love, they soon find themselves in contact with universal love.

Marion began with physical therapy and discovered that emotions were also at work in the body. Her method has now expanded to include the spiritual aspect of the body/mind expression.

> The clue to the work is in the fact that the universe is love. Our loving is then connected to the all-love of the universe. We do not feel lonely but feel part of the universe. Our love goes through a channel to that big love. It is not a love that we hold onto or hold back or that we have for somebody or a thing. It is just love in us that includes everything and everybody around us and goes way beyond ourselves. It has a different quality to it…it is not love that is needy, or to be given only under certain circumstances. It is the kind of love that is always there, that is acknowledged as part of our being.
>
> I'm certain that this is at the bottom of many of the healing processes that go on. When people get into that state, they really allow their body to function. They do not hold back. They do not interfere with their function, they let it totally work. They also have the possibility of letting support come from other places. There's no holding back the love of others, of the universe. There is a give and take just like in the breathing, which is a taking in and a giving out. An attitude of surrender is included which allows this all to happen. You do not oppose the universe, but become part of the universe. Letting this happen is the attitude of surrender and trust.

As you open up, the channel widens. If you hold it back the way is not open; it has been blocked. Sometimes we get a glimpse of it anyway, here and there. But to live in grace you really have to open through that unconditional surrender.

This work brings you to a place where there is no barrier between your internal experience and your external expression of yourself. This is what we call the growth process.

When the diaphragm releases, full inspiration and expiration take place without effort or inhibition. With this "letting go" or "surrender," peace, acceptance and deep love are felt. It is not specific love, but universal love. It shows in the client's face and in his words: "I feel so happy." "I feel so peaceful." "At first I thought I was in love with you, but what I feel is bigger than that." It is important that the practitioner remind the client that it is his capacity for loving that he is feeling; it is universal love and is available to all.

In the moment of surrender, he has gone through a transition. The emergence from that transition is a special moment in the relationship between client and practitioner, known and felt by both. It comes by grace, through allowing and accepting.

8

CONCLUSION

A person is neither a thing nor a process but an opening or a clearing through which the Absolute can manifest.

—Martin Heidegger

What lies behind us and before us are small matters compared to what lies within us.

—Ralph Waldo Emerson

Closing Reflections on Rosen Method

Rosen Method helps the client find his own truth through spontaneous expression. The body supports and confirms the client's story. If the client says something that is not an expression of his true experience, the body does not respond in kind. When the client says what is true—that is, his actual experience of himself—his body responds through relaxation with free movement of the breath. The shift in his consciousness is perceptible in his body.

Much of Rosen Method amounts to following the process closely and slowly, letting the client know when "that's not it" until the client finds his truth. Each shift weakens the hold of habit and new aspects of the person emerge.

The underlying theme in Rosen Method is acceptance. When we teach students to listen deeply and respond, we teach them acceptance in its essential form. Rosen Method uses the body as the channel for this communication.

Our touching is the essence of what we have to say with our hands. We touch tension as the pathway for touching through to essence, saying an unconditional "yes" to everything that arises for the client and an unconditional "yes" to everything that arises in us. Through developing the many skills necessary to become a Rosen Method practitioner, it becomes possible to live life more fully.

Rosen Method is described in the Institute's brochure as "the gateway to awareness through relaxation." There is, however, something beyond relaxation and that is acceptance and grace which is not an active state; rather it is a sense of neutrality and openness to the infinite.

In Rosen Method, the client's story is not fundamental; the underlying goodness, wholeness, essence, or being is fundamental. The practitioner holds the client in her consciousness as *being* and proceeds from there, meeting the person *being* to *being*, rather than relying on technique. The practitioner may see the client's possibilities for wholeness more clearly, but the work is the client's work. Holdings do not remain unconscious; they emerge into the light and become conscious. This work can help one find the core of his being and his connection with all that is.

Appreciation of Marion Rosen

Marion is a physical therapist by training and profession. She is quick to point out that she is not a psychologist, has no training in the field and does not teach psychotherapy.

Her work brings her clients beyond individuality into something more inclusive than the individual and bigger than he is. A practitioner needs to discriminate, to be willing to give up preconceptions in favor of feeling, looking, listening and being open to what is happening in each moment of a session. This Marion does with mastery. Her gifts are extraordinary presence and simplicity.

Experiential knowing, rapt attention and intuitive creativity are the essence of Marion's work. She teaches her students to see and follow the truth as it emerges in a client and to get out of the way in the part of the work where the practitioner cannot participate—the client's shift in consciousness—and thereby to facilitate the client's new possibilities and the experiences of optimum health and well-being.

She sees herself as an educator to whom people come to learn about themselves. When the muscular holding is relaxed, maximum or optimum consciousness can be achieved, resulting in expanded physical, emotional and spiritual well-being.

According to Eastern thought, there is a single root cause of anxiety and that is separation from the inner self. Spiritual practice aims to remedy this separation by bringing one through several stages to unfold the inner being. In this view, connection with self is the only thing that can bring happiness, strength, freedom and the ability to connect wholly with others. Rosen Method offers another path to the same place.

Philosophers and mystics of all cultures have stated that only when we live in contact with the inner self can we be considered to have matured as human beings. Spiritual teachers and philosophers teach that the inner self is identical with the highest truth and that to discover this self within is actually the goal of human life.

The basis of many forms of therapy, spiritual practice and Rosen Method is to move through the layers of accumulated stories, repressed emotions and experiences to touch that which is real in each of us, whether it is called essence, inner self, or being and then to bring that forth in the way we live our lives.

We have what we seek. It is there all the time and if we give it time, it will make itself known to us.

—Thomas Merton

AFTERWORD

When this book was written in 1985 as part of my doctoral dissertation, it was meant to be an aid to students and perhaps of some interest to clients. I was one of eleven students in Marion's first training class. Marion's work came out of her life's experiences as well as her training in physical therapy and relaxation techniques. She did not have many words to describe what she was doing, since from her perspective she was not doing anything except being herself. We watched as she worked and did our best to imitate her. When we asked her what she was doing, she usually said, "doodling." It was clear to me that she was not "doodling;" she was actually doing something that was very effective and which she was doing her best to teach.

I took it upon myself to put into writing what came so naturally to her. It took two years to gather information from her teaching and another three years to compile it into book manuscript form. I would write a chapter and read it to Marion. She would say, "That's it! You've got it!" Then I would write some more and read it to her from the beginning.

Very often she would say, "No, that's not the way it is; you'll have to start over." And so it went for three years until it was finally finished and approved by Marion.

At first, it was photocopied and used as a handout in the classes that came later. At that time, training in what became known as Rosen Method was available only through the newly-formed Rosen Institute in Berkeley. When the intensive training track was developed, training became available well beyond the San Francisco Bay Area and soon my little book was translated and published into Swedish, Finnish, Danish, French and Spanish. I continued to have my book printed in lots of 200 and sold the English language copies myself. When Marion co-authored her own book, coupled with the high cost of printing my book, when the last copies sold, I believed that to be the end of it. With this year marking the 20th anniversary of its publication and with a new growing demand from students, interns, clients and practitioners, I decided to take another look at my book and rethink my decision to let it remain out of print.

In the early years of Rosen Method, the only official training available was through the two-year weekly course that Marion taught with a co-teacher. Marion also offered weekend or five day experiential workshops. Students who attended the workshops again and again often came from afar and could not attend the long-term weekly classes. In an effort to make the training available to those students from out of the area, I, as director of teaching, suggested that we try another format. The teaching group did not think this was a good approach at the time. I then worked to refine what became known as the intensive format and presented the Board of Directors with a proposal for a two year pilot program of ten-day intensives to be held during the summer when the long term training was not in session. My proposal was accepted and in June of 1984 the first Rosen Method intensive was held in Berkeley, with twenty-four students coming from Europe, Scandinavia, Canada and distant places in the U.S. It was a huge success. After the second summer of the pilot program, the intensive program was integrated into the official training offered by the Rosen Institute.

In the early 80's Marion and her niece (who lived in Sweden and who was a student in Marion's first training class) went to Sweden at the invitation of Hans Axelson, the owner and director of a bodywork school in Stockholm. Marion started teaching the five day workshops there and I also taught with her many times. As also happened in Berkeley, people came again and again to the workshops and wanted more than a workshop; they wanted to be fully trained in Rosen Method. One day just before the lunch break, I announced that students who wanted more training could meet with me during lunch around a table in the teaching room. Fifty students showed up and I described the intensive program in Berkeley. They were very excited about it. Hans Axelson agreed to sponsor the program and I was named director of teaching and liaison between Axelsons and the Rosen Institute. The first intensive in Sweden was held at Axelsons in 1986.

The first *residential* intensive was held in Sechelt, B.C., Canada, in 1988, at the invitation of Anne Gregory, who had been a long time student of Marion's. Anne and her husband, Dr. Charles Gregory and I, along with three others, formed the first Board of Directors of the first training center outside the U.S., which was later named the Cascadia Centre. Anne was the administrator and became a teacher in 1994. I was director of teaching and taught along with Anne until 1999, when the center was turned over to others. By introducing a residential component into the intensive format a new and deeper dynamic was set into motion. I returned to Berkeley full of excitement about how powerful the residential intensives were. After two such scenarios Marion was convinced and the teachers' group agreed that Berkeley should offer one too. The first Berkeley sponsored residential intensive was held in Calistoga at the very rustic Rainbow Ranch, until it was transformed a few years ago into the elegant Mayacamas Ranch. We have been meeting there each June since 1990, and it is the only intensive that Marion and I still teach together.

In 1988, when I turned 60, I realized that I had a life full of Rosen Method and very little personal life. I resigned from the Rosen Institute and Gloria Hessellund took my place as director of teaching. Gloria and I had traveled together for many years and introduced Rosen Method in several Scandinavian countries. We were the first teachers to go to Finland and in 1983 taught an introductory workshop that neither of us will ever forget. She also took my place as director of teaching in Sweden while I moved on to Finland to become the director there. Creating a new center is always exciting and I enjoy working intimately with people who want to bring something new and good into their communities. I have also started training centers in Switzerland, France and Holland, each based on an invitation from someone who had training in Rosen Method and who wanted to bring the work to their area. After a few introductory workshops, enough interest is generated to start offering intensives. My goal in starting training centers has been to stay on as director until it is self-sustaining, training local teachers who will teach in the local language and who will later become the director of their center. I move on and start another center. It gives me great pleasure to return as a visiting teacher to meet people that I have known over many years and to see how they have made the work their own and how much their lives have changed through the work. The willingness to persevere through the difficult process of start-up comes from a love of Rosen Method and a conviction that this work can make a positive difference in people's lives and ultimately in the world around them.

When the intensive program was first approved by the Rosen Institute, Marion and I taught all of the intensives together (excepting Canada) to make sure that students could be successfully trained and certified through this format and to also make sure that the Rosen Method training standards could be upheld. After we taught eleven intensives together and were well satisfied that it was possible, we taught three more for good measure before separating so that we could train other teachers to teach in the intensive format. Now that there are five training centers with two more on the way in the U.S. and ten centers in other countries, Marion and I rarely teach together.

My goal has always been to codify Marion's work so that it could be passed on to others in a structured and coherent fashion, doing my best to leave room for each individual to find his or her personal expression of the work. As teachers, we created lists of requirements and time frames, lists of what must be learned and lists of rules and regulations. I often wonder now if by creating such tight parameters we have taken the aliveness and spontaneity out of the process. Rosen Method is Marion's unique expression of herself and her life's experiences and training. She does not practice Rosen Method; rather, she approaches each client as Marion Rosen, and she does what only she can do. The rest of us do our best to take what we have learned from her and our teachers, making the work a unique expression of ourselves, doing what only we can do, while staying within a framework of that which can be identified as Rosen Method.

Although Rosen Method is a dynamic, organic process, its fundamental principles, as outlined in this book, are as true today as when they were first written. I have been practicing and teaching Rosen Method since 1979. I have noticed some changes in the work itself and many changes in the way it is taught. The original emphasis was in following the client's process to where the source of holding and the emotion beneath the holding came into awareness. As the holding softened and the emotion was expressed, we considered the process complete, although we acknowledged that there was now more energy for living and more movement and breath in the body, along with possibilities for self actualization in the client's life.

My expression of Rosen Method in my practice and in my teaching has become one of reaching through or beyond the client's tension in such a way that he can feel himself *as the person he was meant to be.* When a client remembers who he is, his life changes. I am more interested in what is possible than in what happened, although often both surface. Often, one has to go through what happened in order to reclaim what is possible. I notice that a box of tissues in my office lasts a very long time nowadays. There are far fewer tears now and more joy and peace that clients discover in themselves.

It has long been my goal to make Rosen Method bigger than what we do at the table one hour at a time by using the principles of Rosen Method for living an authentic life. My current passion in my professional life is working with interns. I work with interns privately as well as in an intern group, since the internship is often a lonely and daunting time and most interns want to be in some kind of a supportive group during this time. My supervision group was created casually by the interns and began just as many training centers have begun: "If we get together and find a place, will you come?" From there it has evolved into daylong supervision marathons at my house each month whenever possible and a two or three day overnight retreat every four months or so. Some teachers and practitioners also attend the intern gatherings and experience the teaching as a form of continuing education.

In my work with interns, I make the internship a true apprenticeship. I accept as interns only those with whom I feel I can have a close personal relationship, who I think have the potential for becoming excellent practitioners and who will stay with the process for as long as it takes. We make this agreement before we begin. From that point on, we work together, developing a relationship based on loyalty, trust and intimacy. I am available to interns whenever their questions arise. Although I recognize the value of meeting the requirements for certification and ticking them off within the required time frame, that is not my primary concern. Most of my interns are excited by this approach and appreciate the "readiness" factor. I look for authenticity in each intern so that the person he or she is in daily life is the person who comes to the table to give sessions. Ticking off the list of requirements does not equal certification.

Editing this book after twenty years has served to remind me of all that I have "learned" and now "know" about the profound simplicity of this deep inner work as a pathway to transformation—in Marion's words, "from the person we think we are to the person we really are. In the end, we cannot be anyone else."

Rosen Method and Marion Rosen herself have enriched my life enormously. Working with interns as I do is my way of giving back for all that I have received. To play my part in training practitioners who bring honor to Marion's work in their practice and in their lives is a great privilege.

—Elaine L. Mayland, Ph.D.

ABOUT THE AUTHOR

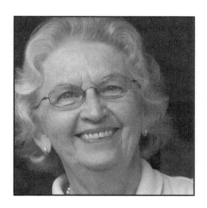

Elaine L. Mayland has a Ph.D. in transpersonal psychology. She developed the intensive training program through the Rosen Institute in Berkeley, California, making Rosen Method available to students around the world, and is also the founder of several training centers. She continues to teach Rosen Method and has a private practice in Palo Alto, California.